NEUROPSYCHOPHARMACOLOGY AND THE AFFECTIVE DISORDERS

NEW ENGLAND JOURNAL OF MEDICINE
MEDICAL PROGRESS SERIES

NEUROPSYCHOPHARMACOLOGY AND THE AFFECTIVE DISORDERS

JOSEPH J. SCHILDKRAUT, M.D.
ASSISTANT PROFESSOR OF PSYCHIATRY,
HARVARD MEDICAL SCHOOL;
DIRECTOR, NEUROPSYCHOPHARMACOLOGY LABORATORY,
MASSACHUSETTS MENTAL HEALTH CENTER,
BOSTON

LITTLE, BROWN AND COMPANY
BOSTON

LIBRARY OF CONGRESS CATALOG CARD NO. 71–112012
4176-15D2-M07/70
FIRST EDITION

THIS MONOGRAPH FIRST APPEARED AS A SERIES OF MEDICAL PROGRESS REPORTS IN THE NEW ENGLAND JOURNAL OF MEDICINE. PUBLICATION IN BOOK FORM INCORPORATES ADDITIONAL MATERIAL AND ILLUSTRATIONS.

Published in Great Britain
by J. & A. Churchill, London

British Standard Book No. 7000 0185 9

PRINTED IN THE UNITED STATES OF AMERICA

To BETSY, PETER, SIMON, SHIRLEY

PREFACE

IN recent years drugs have become available for the treatment of some types of depressions and manias, i.e., the major affective disorders. The biochemical pharmacology of these and related psychoactive drugs has been studied extensively in the hope of uncovering clues to explain the chemical mechanisms by which these drugs alter mood in man. These studies have provided substantial evidence to suggest that the biogenic amines (namely, the catecholamines norepinephrine and dopamine, and the indoleamine serotonin) may be of importance.

This book reviews the findings of the past decade on the changes in biogenic amine metabolism produced by various psychoactive drugs. These include amphetamine and cocaine, which are stimulants or euphoriants; the monoamine oxidase inhibitors and tricyclic (imipramine-like) compounds, which are antidepressants; reserpine, which may cause depressions; and lithium salts, which have recently generated considerable public interest because of their efficacy in the treatment of mania.

In addition to suggesting possible mechanisms of action by which these drugs may exert their clinical effects on affective state, neuropharmacologic findings have suggested heuristic hypotheses concerning the possible biochemical changes that may occur in depressions or manias. Such hypotheses have prompted the study of biogenic amine metabolism in patients with affective disorders, and the findings are described in this report.

Also emphasized is the importance of differentiating among the various depressive syndromes when one selects the appropriate treatment for a depressed patient. Clinical criteria for diagnosing endogenous, schizoaffective, chronic characterologic and situational depressions are outlined, and suggestions are provided for treatment. Discussion of the treatment of the endogenous depressions incorporates neuropharmacologic and neurochemical concepts into the suggestions for clinical management.

Since the contents of this book originally appeared in the *New England Journal of Medicine,* sections have been revised and new material has been added on differential diagnosis and treatment of the depressive disorders and contraindications and side effects of the major antidepressant drugs.

This book is directed to the psychiatrist and any other physician who must diagnose and treat patients with affective disorders. It is also intended for the basic scientist concerned with the effects of drugs on neurochemistry and behavior, and for the medical student in the hope that it will aid in the transition from course work in neuropharmacology to clinical work in psychiatry.

I am grateful for the many helpful comments on this manuscript that I received from Dr. Franz J. Ingelfinger of the *New England Journal of Medicine,* as well as from many of my colleagues. I also thank Miss Sheila Eder and Mrs. Donna Graham, who typed part of the manuscript and provided valuable assistance in compiling the references.

Although I am indebted to all the many investigators whose work is summarized in this volume, I specifically want to acknowledge my own principal research collaborators, Drs. Jack Durell, Gerald L. Klerman, Irwin J. Kopin and Saul M. Schanberg, each of whom has contributed significantly to this field. I am particularly grateful to Dr. Milton Greenblatt for initially stimulating my interest in this area of research, and to Dr. Seymour S. Kety for the critical judgment and enthusiasm that he provided while I was a member of his laboratory and thereafter as well. Above all, I express my appreciation to Dr. Jack R. Ewalt, Bullard Professor of Psychiatry, Harvard Medical School, who has consistently given his unfailing counsel and generous support throughout the past ten years.

J. J. S.

Boston

CONTENTS

INTRODUCTION

DURING the past decade, a number of drugs have been found to be effective in the treatment of affective disorders (depressions and manias), and these drugs have been shown to alter the metabolism and the physiologic activity of the biogenic amines (norepinephrine, dopamine and serotonin), both in animals and in man. Almost invariably, drugs that affect one of these amines will alter the metabolism of another, and it has been difficult to isolate these effects experimentally, suggesting that functionally important interactions of the biogenic amines may occur within the brain. These could occur as a result of either common chemical and pharmacologic properties of the monoamines or the neuroanatomical interconnections of the monoaminergic neuronal systems (for example, synaptic connections between noradrenergic and serotonergic neurons).

Despite some discrepancies, most data seem compatible with the hypothesis that drugs which elevate mood may increase one or another of the biogenic amines at receptor sites in brain, whereas drugs that cause depressions or are effective in the treatment of manias may decrease the activity of monoamines at receptors. Correspondingly, studies of biogenic amine metabolism in patients with affective disorders suggest that deficiencies of norepinephrine or serotonin may occur in at least some types of depressions, whereas elations may be associated with an excess of one or another of the monoamines.

Although only tentative conclusions may be drawn from the findings at present, the recent increase in research activity in this area attests to the heuristic value of these hypotheses. Considerable further investigation will thus be required to explore the leads provided by contemporary studies. But the progress of the past decade suggests that, in the case of the affective disorders, pharmacology may ultimately provide a critical bridge between neurochemistry and clinical psychiatry.*

* Schildkraut, J. J. Rationale of some approaches used in biochemical studies of the affective disorders: The pharmacological bridge. In *Psychochemical Research in Man: Methods, Strategy and Theory*. Edited by A. J. Mandell and M. P. Mandell. New York: Academic, 1969. Pp. 113–126.

NEUROPSYCHOPHARMACOLOGY AND THE AFFECTIVE DISORDERS

1

CLASSIFICATION OF THE AFFECTIVE DISORDERS

DRUGS that are clinically effective in the treatment of the affective disorders — depressions and manias — have also been found to be important tools for research in psychiatry during the past decade.[1-17] Since these disorders, particularly the depressions, represent a heterogeneous collection of entities, their differential diagnosis and classification have occasioned a long-standing controversy.[17a-19] A preliminary discussion of the diagnosis and classifications of the affective disorders is necessary, therefore, if the action of the agents developed to treat them is to be understood.

The term *depression* as it is commonly used in clinical psychiatry may refer to a mood state that is within the normal range, a pathologic symptom, one or more clinical syndromes or one or more diseases. As a normal mood, depression refers to the affective state of sadness which occurs in a wide variety of human situations, such as grief and mourning or disappointment and failure. The relation of this normal mood to the pathologic mood disorders has not been extensively studied. Depression as a pathologic symptom of sadness of affect is differentiated from the normal mood by the intensity, duration or quality of the affective state. As a symptom, depression is found in a variety of clinical disorders, only some of which are primarily psychiatric.

Depression may also refer to one or more syndromes,

or clusterings of symptoms: sadness of affect; crying; feelings of hopelessness, helplessness, worthlessness and guilt; suicidal preoccupations; loss of drive and ambition; fatigue; psychic retardation; motor retardation or agitation; anxiety; sleep disturbance; loss of appetite; weight loss; constipation; and diurnal fluctuation of symptoms. The term *depression* may also be used to designate one or more putative disease entities. Although the notion of the depressions as a group of biologically discrete diseases has considerable historical precedent and is maintained by many biologically oriented investigators, there are, as yet, relatively few biologic data upon which to base a meaningful classification of these disorders.[20]

Appropriate clinical subgroupings of the depressions have long been sought, and a number of clinical dichotomies (such as "endogenous-reactive," "neurotic-psychotic" or "retarded-agitated") have been suggested for classifying the depressions. Although these groupings have had some limited value in biologic studies, it is unlikely that any simple dichotomous separation will be adequate to classify the depressions into biologically meaningful subgroups, and many more complex classifications have also been suggested.[19,21–29] For example, the current diagnostic manual of the American Psychiatric Association (APA) differentiates among manic-depressive disorders, involutional melancholias, schizoaffective depressions, psychotic depressive reactions and depressive neuroses.[29]

In the APA classification, the various subtypes of the manic-depressive illnesses (defined therein to include cases that are exclusively mania or depression) and involutional melancholia comprise the "major affective disorders."[29] Correspondingly, these "major" depressive disorders have been designated as the "endogenous depressions" in other systems of classification,[28,30] but in some systems, involutional melancholia is not included among the "endogenous depressions." [31] The "manic-depressive depressions," as defined in the APA classification, may comprise a number of genetically distinct entities.[32–34] Some classifications, therefore, restrict the term *manic-depressive* to cyclical mood disorders in which there is a history of at least one attack of a manic as well as a depressive episode; endogenous depressions occurring in the absence of a history of mania are separately classified (see Table 1, below).[28] The APA classification states that the onset of the "major affective disorders" does not seem to be related directly to a precipitating life experience.[29] Some investigators, including me, however, think that more relevant distinguishing characteristics of these ("major" or "endogenous") depressions are the autonomy of the depression once it is established and the lack of reactivity of the symptoms either to day-to-day alterations in the patient's environment or to interpersonal treatment modalities.[28]

According to the APA classification, the "manic-depressive depressions" are subject to remissions and recurrences, and "are characterized by severely depressed mood and by mental and motor retardation"; many investigators have similarly stressed the retardation, as well as the clear delineation of the depressive interval in the endogenous depressions. Involutional melancholia is further described as "a disorder occurring in the involutional period and characterized by worry, anxiety, agitation and severe insomnia," frequently with "feelings of guilt and somatic preoccupation which may be of delusional proportions." [29] Schizoaffective depressions, psychotic depressive reactions and depressive neuroses are defined and grouped separately from the "major affective disorders" in the recent APA classification (Table 1).[29] Similarly, in the system of classification that I use, schizoaffective depressions, chronic characterologic de-

TABLE 1. *Classifications of the Depressions*

APA CLASSIFICATION (ABBREVIATED)

I. Major affective disorders
  A. Manic-depressive illnesses
    1. Manic-depressive, circular
    2. Manic-depressive, depressed
  B. Involutional melancholias
II. Schizoaffective disorders
III. Psychotic depressive reactions
IV. Depressive neuroses

MY CLASSIFICATION

I. Endogenous depressions
  A. Manic-depressive depressions
  B. Recurrent depressions
  C. Nonrecurrent depressions
  D. Involutional melancholias
II. Schizoaffective depressions
III. Chronic characterologic depressions
IV. Situational depressions

pressions and situational depressions are separated from the endogenous depressions.[28] (Table 1; cf. Chapter 6) It is possible that some of these disorders are segments of a continuum rather than distinct nosologic entities, but this change in conceptual framework does not alter the finding that differences between the various groupings of depressed patients are meaningful and may be therapeutically relevant distinctions.[19,20]

The classifications of the depressions devised thus far are, at best, preliminary and limited solutions to a major problem in psychiatry. Whereas many cases may be uniquely classified according to these systems, an appreciable number will fall within the ill-defined areas separating one or another of the groups or subgroups. With this awareness, however, attention has been focused on these systems of classification, and the separation of the "major affective disorders" or "endogenous depressions" from other depressions is stressed. This has been done since separation of the different types of depressions, I believe, is of considerable importance, both when the appropriate course of treatment for a depressed patient is under consideration and when the results of clinical pharmacologic or biochemical studies of patients with affective disorders are interpreted (see Chapter 6).

2

ANTIDEPRESSANTS AND OTHER DRUGS USED CLINICALLY

THE three classes of drugs most commonly used in the treatment of depressive disorders are the psychomotor stimulants (of which amphetamine is the prototype), the monoamine oxidase inhibitors and the tricyclic antidepressants (that is, imipramine and its congeners). It is of some historical interest that cocaine, which was recognized as a stimulant and euphoriant by Freud,[35] may be regarded as the forerunner of the modern antidepressant drugs with which it shares many neuropharmacologic properties. The problem of addiction limited the clinical investigation of cocaine in depression, and the systematic use of stimulant drugs in the treatment of depressions began with the use of amphetamine in the 1930's.[36,37] It was not until the introduction of the monoamine oxidase inhibitors and the tricyclic antidepressants a little more than 10 years ago, however, that the era of effective pharmacologic therapy of depressions began.[38–40] Despite the efficacy of these antidepressant drugs, electroconvulsive therapy still remains the most effective form of treatment for some depressed patients.[41]

Amphetamine and Other Psychomotor Stimulants

The psychomotor stimulants (for example, amphetamine, methamphetamine and methylphenidate) cause mood elevation, increased alertness and enhanced performance in normal subjects.[42,43] These drugs may alleviate some of the symptoms of depression in certain depressed patients, but such beneficial effects are often transient and may be accompanied by a number of unwanted side effects. A review of the clinical pharmacology of these compounds may be found elsewhere.[2,42] It is fairly generally agreed that the psychomotor stimulants have relatively little to offer in the treatment of the major depressive disorders.[1,2,5,7] These drugs, however, may prove to be of some value experimentally, in separating the various types of depressive disorders. For example, in one study, after the acute administration of methamphetamine, patients with the diagnosis of "neurotic depression"* were found to have a euphoric response, whereas patients with "psychotic depressions"* experienced dysphoria.[44] Recent preliminary findings suggest also that the response to d-amphetamine may be useful in predicting the clinical response to imipramine in depressed patients.[45]

Monoamine Oxidase Inhibitors

The monoamine oxidase inhibitor antidepressants, as their name suggests, inhibit the activity of the enzyme monoamine oxidase.[13,46] Iproniazid, a hydrazine derivative, was the first compound of this class that was shown to be effective in the treatment of depressive disorders.[38,39] Because of the serious hepatotoxicity associated with the use of this drug in some patients, other monoamine oxidase inhibitors have been introduced during

* Since these diagnoses were not made according to the classifications discussed above, the interested reader may wish to consult the paper[44] for the diagnostic criteria used in this study.

the past decade; these include phenelzine, isocarboxazid and nialamide (which are hydrazine derivatives), as well as tranylcypromine and pargyline* (which are nonhydrazine compounds).

The clinical effectiveness of the monoamine oxidase inhibitors in the treatment of depressive disorders has been studied fairly extensively over the past decade.[1,2,5,7] Although there are many inconsistencies among the numerous investigations, a recent evaluation of the double-blind controlled studies in the literature suggested that iproniazid, phenelzine and tranylcypromine were clinically effective antidepressant compounds for at least certain depressed patients;[1] this conclusion was reached independently by other reviewers.[2] It has been suggested that one or another specific group of depressed patients may be particularly responsive to treatment with the monoamine oxidase inhibitors,[47,48] but this hypothesis requires further documentation.

Selective responsivity of some, but not all, depressed patients to treatment with monoamine oxidase inhibitors could account for the discrepancies in findings of various studies, since the clinical population of most studies has included a heterogeneous group of depressed patients. Because of the variability of clinical response and the possibility of toxic side effects, including the hypertensive cerebrovascular reactions that can occur in patients treated with monoamine oxidase inhibitors upon ingestion of foods containing sympathomimetic amines or their precursors[2] (cf. Appendix II), these agents are generally not recommended as the first drug to be prescribed in the treatment of most depressed patients.

* Pargyline is currently available for the treatment of hypertension.

Tricyclic Antidepressants

The successful treatment of depressions with imipramine, the prototype of the tricyclic antidepressants,* was first described by Kuhn[40] a little more than 10 years ago. Since that time, a number of other tricyclic antidepressants have been developed; these include desmethylimipramine (a demethylated derivative of imipramine), amitriptyline, nortriptyline (demethylated amitriptyline) and protriptyline.

The clinical antidepressant activity of imipramine and amitriptyline has been fairly well substantiated by a number of double-blind controlled studies.[1] Although the other tricyclic antidepressants have been studied less extensively, available evidence suggests that they are efficacious.[1] The clinical pharmacologic differences between the various tricyclic antidepressants are, generally, of less importance than their similarities. Amitriptyline, the most sedative of these compounds, may be particularly useful in the treatment of agitated depressions, whereas tricyclic antidepressants that are less sedating may be more suitable in retarded depressions,[2,5] but further controlled studies will be required to test these impressions.

All these drugs require prolonged administration (usually one to four weeks) before antidepressant effects may be observed, and this is a limitation in their usefulness, particularly in the treatment of the suicidal patient. Little clinical evidence supports the prediction, made on the basis of studies in animals, that the demethylated congeners (such as desmethylimipramine) might act more rapidly than the parent compounds.[2]

In his initial report on the treatment of depressions

* The designation *tricyclic antidepressants* refers to the chemical ring structure common to this class of drugs (cf. Appendix III).

with imipramine, Kuhn[40] stressed the importance of the differential diagnosis of the depressive disorders when physicians prescribe this drug. Imipramine, Kuhn asserted, was "primarily indicated and effective in the treatment of endogenous depressions," which were described as showing "typical symptoms of mental and motor retardation, fatigue, feelings of heaviness, hopelessness, guilt and despair," as well as "aggravation of symptoms in the morning with a tendency to improvement during the day." [40] This observation has been confirmed in some controlled studies,[41,49] but not in all.[50] Kuhn also noted that imipramine could lead to an exacerbation of the psychosis in schizophrenic patients and that it might intensify an episode of mania in manic-depressive patients. These findings have been confirmed, and similar observations have been made during treatment with monoamine oxidase inhibitors.[2] Mild, transient, self-limited, hypomanic symptomatology is almost invariably observed in patients with endogenous depressions during the course of treatment with imipramine.[51]

More recent observations[41] further emphasize the need for differentiating among the depressions when one is deciding on appropriate treatment. When patients are treated in a hospital setting, the placebo response rate of various depressions may differ markedly; thus, certain types of depressions (for example, "neurotic"* or "character disorder"*) may be adequately treated by interpersonal technics without pharmacologically active drugs. In contrast, the comparatively low placebo response rate found in "manic-depressive"* or "involutional"* depressions[41] supports the need for somatic therapy in the treatment of these disorders. Failure to differentiate among the types of depression and the inclusion in some clinical drug evaluations of patients either with disor-

* The diagnostic criteria used in this study are specified elsewhere.[41]

ders having high placebo response rates or with disorders for which the drug might otherwise be contraindicated (such as schizophrenia) may account for some of the discrepant findings in the many studies of the clinical efficacy of the tricyclic antidepressants.

Various phenothiazines (for example, chlorpromazine and thioridazine), which are structurally related to the tricyclic antidepressants (cf. Appendix III), have been reported as effective in the treatment of certain depressive disorders in some but not all studies.[52–55] Phenothiazines, however, do not seem to be effective in patients with "retarded depressions,"* whereas tricyclic antidepressants are most effective in this group.[53]

Lithium Salts

Lithium salts have come to occupy an important place in the treatment of affective disorders — particularly hypomania and mania.[3] These agents, however, must be distinguished from the antidepressant drugs. The therapeutic efficacy of lithium salts in the treatment of mania was first reported 20 years ago[56] and has been fairly well established since that time.[3] More recently, it has been suggested that lithium salts might exert a prophylactic action in the treatment of recurrent manic-depressive disorders and also in the recurrent depressions in which no manic episode occurs.[3,57] The efficacy of lithium salts in the prophylactic treatment of manic-depressive disorders, however, has been questioned.[58] Lithium salts, when administered during the depressed phase of major affective disorders, appear to be relatively ineffective as

* Disorders so classified in this study[53] may be included under the classification of the "major" or "endogenous" depressions described in Chapters 1 and 6.

antidepressant agents, although occasional reports of an antidepressant action may be found.[3,59] At present, the effectiveness of lithium salts seems well documented only in the treatment of hypomania and mania.[3]*

* Lithium carbonate has recently been approved by the F.D.A. for use in treatment of the manic phase of manic-depressive disorders.

3

NEUROPHARMACOLOGIC STUDIES OF DRUGS USED CLINICALLY

SINCE the initial observation that reserpine, a drug that could cause depressions in some patients, depletes the brain of various biogenic amines in animals, whereas the monoamine oxidase inhibitor antidepressants increase levels of biogenic amines in the central nervous system, the effects of these and other psychoactive drugs on biogenic amine metabolism have been extensively studied. The catecholamines, norepinephrine and dopamine, and the indoleamine, serotonin, are the brain monoamines that have received the greatest attention. Norepinephrine is present in many areas of the brain, but it is most highly concentrated in the hypothalamus; norepinephrine also occurs in the peripheral sympathetic nervous system.[60-63] Dopamine is most highly concentrated in the basal ganglia; in other areas of the brain it occurs in much lower concentrations.[62,63] Although found in high concentration in various peripheral tissues, serotonin is also present in the brain in appreciable amounts.[60,63-66] The regional distribution of the biogenic amines in brain has been extensively studied by recently developed histochemical fluorescence technics, and specific monoamine-containing neurons have been described.[67,68] High densities of these neurons occur in the hypothalamus and limbic system — brain structures that may be important in affective states.

Although it is generally accepted that norepinephrine

functions as a chemical transmitter in the peripheral sympathetic nervous system,[61] such a function for this and other amines in the central nervous system has not yet been clarified. It has been suggested that norepinephrine, dopamine, serotonin and possibly other biogenic amines may each serve as a transmitter substance at one or another synapse in the central nervous system, or that one or more of them may modulate or regulate synaptic transmission possibly mediated by another chemical transmitter, for example, acetylcholine.[69,70]

Most of our understanding of norepinephrine metabolism comes from studies of peripheral sympathetic nerves; but similar, although not necessarily identical, pathways of metabolism appear to occur in the brain.[9] Norepinephrine is synthesized in the neuron from the amino acid tyrosine through the intermediates 3,4-dihydroxyphenylalanine (dopa) and dopamine; it is then stored in intraneuronal granules. Norepinephrine, discharged from neuronal endings in physiologically active form either by nerve impulses or by sympathomimetic drugs, is thought to be inactivated mainly by neuronal re-uptake or by enzymatic conversion by catechol O-methyl transferase to normetanephrine. Norepinephrine released intracellularly, either spontaneously or by pharmacologic interference with the binding mechanism (as by reserpine-like drugs), appears to be inactivated by mitochondrial monoamine oxidase before leaving the cell, with formation of the deaminated catechol metabolites, 3,4-dihydroxymandelic acid and 3,4-dihydroxyphenyl glycol. Monoamine oxidase may thus regulate tissue levels of norepinephrine without necessarily acting to terminate the physiologic activity of norepinephrine at the receptor. Levels of normetanephrine may reflect the level of norepinephrine discharged extraneuronally onto adrenergic receptors[71–77] (Figs. 1–3).

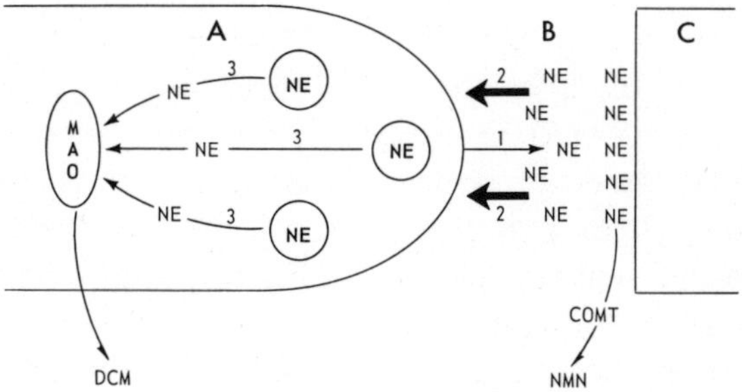

FIGURE 1. *Noradrenergic Neuron and Receptor. In this schematic representation of a noradrenergic nerve ending* (A), *synaptic cleft* (B) *and receptor* (C), *NE indicates norepinephrine, NMN normetanephrine, DCM deaminated catechol metabolites, COMT catechol-O-methyl transferase, MAO monoamine oxidase (within a mitochondrion), 1 discharge of norepinephrine into the synaptic cleft and onto receptor, 2 reuptake of norepinephrine from the synaptic cleft, and 3 intracellular release of norepinephrine from storage granules into cytoplasm and onto mitochondrial monoamine oxidase. (From Schildkraut and Kety,* Science *156:21–30, April 7, 1967. Copyright 1967 by the American Association for the Advancement of Science.)*

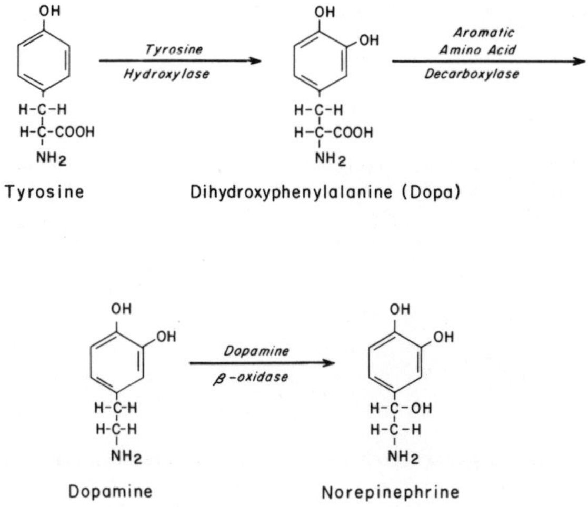

FIGURE 2. *Biosynthesis of Catecholamines.*

Secondary O-methylation or deamination reactions involved in the formation of 3-methoxy-4-hydroxymandelic acid (VMA) or 3-methoxy-4-hydroxyphenylglycol (MHPG) can occur, depending on species, in the central nervous system as well as in the liver or kidney. Most MHPG present in urine is conjugated with sulfate.[78-81] The sulfate conjugate of MHPG has recently been identified in rat brain as a major metabolite of norepinephrine and normetanephrine,[82] and studies of the origin of urinary MHPG support this finding[81] (Fig. 3).

Serotonin is synthesized in the neuron from tryptophan, which is first hydroxylated by the enzyme tryptophan hydroxylase to form 5-hydroxytryptophan. Decarboxylation of 5-hydroxytryptophan produces serotonin, which is stored in the neuron. Serotonin is metabolized by monoamine oxidase, forming 5-hydroxyindoleacetic acid (5HIAA) or 5-hydroxytryptophol.[83-88] Recent evi-

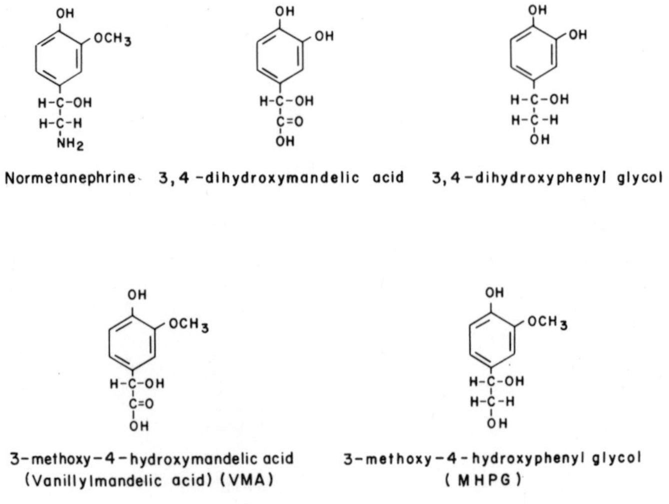

FIGURE 3. *Metabolites of Norepinephrine.*

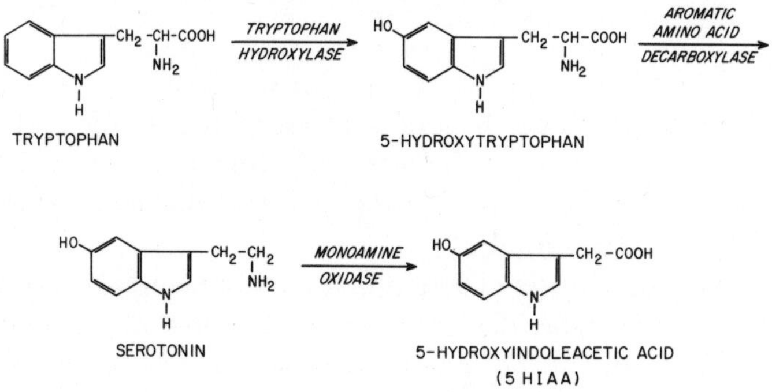

FIGURE 4. *Biosynthesis and Metabolism of Serotonin.*

dence suggests that a mechanism for the neuronal reuptake of serotonin (as exists for norepinephrine) may occur in the brain[89,90] (Fig. 4).

Reserpine and Reserpine-like Drugs

Reserpine, at present, occupies a relatively minor place in the clinical treatment of the affective disorders, but the pharmacology of reserpine and reserpine-like agents is of considerable theoretical interest. Over a decade ago, it was observed that depressions occurred in some patients during treatment with reserpine.[91–94] Remission of the depression generally occurred when reserpine was discontinued, but in some cases electroconvulsive therapy or other forms of treatment were required. Reserpine-induced depressions have been regarded by most clinicians as clinically indistinguishable from certain naturally occurring depressive disorders, although this view has been questioned.[95,96] Depressions occur in only a comparatively small fraction of patients treated with reserpine, and drug dosage may be an important factor;[16,93] hypertensive patients may be particularly susceptible.[96] Many other biochemical, physiologic and psychologic determinants may be involved in reserpine-induced depressions, but this possibility has not been well studied. In animals, reserpine induces a syndrome of behavioral changes, including sedation, which has been proposed as a possible pharmacologic model for depression in man.[97]

By a mechanism of action that has not been fully elucidated, reserpine depletes neuronal stores of biogenic amines, both in peripheral sites and in the brain.[98-101] The capacity of the neuron to bind and store biogenic amines is impaired by reserpine. Norepinephrine synthesis may also be decreased by reserpine, presumably as a result of the reduced accumulation of the precursor, dopamine, in storage granules where the conversion to norepinephrine normally occurs.[102-104] Depletion of norepinephrine, dopamine and serotonin levels in the brain occurs during reserpine-induced sedation. Considerable research has been devoted to the attempt to establish a causal connection between the behavioral effects and the changes in levels of one or another of these amines. The sedative effect of reserpine, however, is not well correlated with the gross level of any one of these monoamines in the brain.[105] In a recent study of a series of reserpine analogues, sedation appeared to be associated with depletion of serotonin rather than catecholamines.[106] Only limited conclusions may be drawn from such measurements of total monoamine levels in brain, however, since physiologic function may depend upon the monoamine content in one or another small but specifically localized (functional) pool.[105,107] After treatment with reserpine, the restoration of the capacity of central neurons to accumulate biogenic amines appears to be correlated with the disappearance of the reserpine-induced sedation.[108,109]

The amino acid precursors of these biogenic amines, unlike the amines themselves, can cross the blood-brain barrier, and they have been used to increase the content of the derivative monoamines in the brain of the reserpine-treated animal.[110] Administration of dopa, the catecholamine precursor, reverses reserpine-induced sedation in animals and restores gross behavior and the conditioned avoidance response to approximately normal levels. The serotonin precursor, 5-hydroxytryptophan, in contrast, does not effectively reverse the impairment of motor performance produced by reserpine in animals, although this amino acid may cause a diffuse, apparently uncoordinated increase in motor activity.[110–114] In a similar study of human subjects, dopa was reported to counteract the psychologic effects of reserpine.[115] On the basis of these observations, some investigators have suggested that catecholamine depletion is of major importance in reserpine-induced sedation in animals and possibly in reserpine-induced depressions in man. But these studies using precursor amino acids must be interpreted cautiously, since the distribution of an amine formed from an exogenously administered precursor is not necessarily identical with the distribution of the endogenous amine.[112,116,117] Moreover, these precursor amino acids may have pharmacologic effects in addition to those resulting from the physiologic actions of the derivative biogenic amines.

Drugs that inhibit the synthesis of norepinephrine or serotonin have also been used to investigate the relation of the various biogenic amines to reserpine-induced sedation. Catecholamine synthesis in the brain may be inhibited by α-methylparatyrosine, an agent that interferes with the enzymatic conversion of tyrosine to dopa; dopamine and norepinephrine levels may thereby be reduced without alterations in serotonin content.[118] When catecholamine synthesis is interrupted by α-methylparatyrosine in animals, sedation or impairment of behavior in a variety of experimental situations has been observed.[118,119] In contrast, sedation is not seen when the enzymatic hydroxylation of tryptophan is inhibited by parachlorophenylalanine, and levels of serotonin in brain are markedly reduced by this drug (without changes in norepinephrine content). After reserpine administration, however, animals in which a large fraction of brain serotonin was previously depleted by parachlorophenylalanine became sedated.[120] These findings have been interpreted to imply that depletion of catecholamines, rather than serotonin, is of importance in the syndrome of reserpine-induced sedation, but, since serotonin is not totally depleted by parachlorophenylalanine, other interpretations of the data are possible.[121]

Other investigators have stressed the role of serotonin in the reserpine syndrome.[108,121] It has been suggested that impairment of amine binding by reserpine does not decrease, but rather increases, the free (unbound) serotonin available to interact with receptor sites in brain, and that this increase in serotonin at receptors accounts for reserpine-induced sedation. This position has been questioned by some;[122] the controversy remains unresolved.

Monoamine Oxidase Inhibitors

The changes in biogenic amine metabolism and the alterations in behavior produced by the monoamine oxidase inhibitors have been studied fairly extensively in animals.[13] In a variety of species treated with monoamine oxidase inhibitors, elevated levels of catecholamines and serotonin in brain have been observed together with increases in behavioral activity.

The behavioral hyperactivity produced by the monoamine oxidase inhibitors in animals has been interpreted as a possible analogue of the antidepressant action of these drugs in man, but it is obvious that such an analogy must be drawn with extreme caution. Inhibition of the enzymatic inactivation of the biogenic amines by monoamine oxidase is assumed to account for the increased levels of monoamines in the brain. As with reserpine, attempts to relate the behavioral changes produced by monoamine oxidase inhibitors to alterations in the metabolism of a specific amine have led to discrepant findings.[13,107] In clinical studies, monoamine oxidase inhibitors have been shown to decrease the urinary excretion of the deaminated metabolites of both norepinephrine and serotonin.[123-125]

In one series of studies in animals[126,127] monoamine oxidase inhibitors were administered to a number of different species. No behavioral excitation occurred in the species in which there was an increase in levels of serotonin without a rise in levels of norepinephrine in brain. In species in which both norepinephrine and serotonin were elevated, behavioral excitation was temporally correlated with higher levels of norepinephrine. These data suggested that the excitation produced by monoamine oxidase inhibitors may result from the spillover of norepinephrine onto receptor sites.[126,127] But in another study, after administration of an amino acid precursor of the catecholamines, dopa, to animals previously treated with a monoamine oxidase inhibitor, the resulting behavioral excitation was better correlated with levels of dopamine than with the level of norepinephrine in the brain.[128] Other studies, however, including one that used the technic of inhibiting monoamine synthesis, have reported the behavioral changes induced by some monoamine oxidase inhibitors to be related to serotonin levels in brain.[129,130]

Monoamine oxidase inhibitors counteract or prevent

reserpine-induced sedation in animals. Numerous studies have shown that, when reserpine is administered to animals previously treated with a monoamine oxidase inhibitor, increased behavioral activity (rather than sedation) is observed.[114,126,127,129,131–133] In most studies the reversal of reserpine-induced sedation by monoamine oxidase inhibitors appears better correlated with alterations in brain norepinephrine or dopamine than with changes in serotonin, but not all investigators have observed this relation.

Tricyclic Antidepressants

Tricyclic antidepressant drugs potentiate the peripheral effects of norepinephrine and serotonin in animals under a wide variety of physiologic conditions.[6,14,134–137] At extremely high doses, however, tricyclic antidepressants may block rather than potentiate the effects of these amines in animals. In man the pressor response to norepinephrine infusion is markedly increased after treatment with imipramine[138,139] or protriptyline.[140] On the basis of the potentiation of the peripheral responses to norepinephrine, it was suggested that "sensitization of central adrenergic synapses" might account for the antidepressant actions of imipramine.[141] Direct evidence to support the assumption that tricyclic antidepressants potentiate norepinephrine in the brain as they do in the periphery, however, is lacking.

A possible mechanism for the potentiation of norepinephrine by tricyclic antidepressants is provided by the finding that imipramine interferes with the uptake of norepinephrine into peripheral and central noradrenergic neurons.[142,143] By inhibiting the neuronal reuptake of norepinephrine, imipramine may prevent the physiologic inactivation of this amine at the synapse, thus causing an increase in levels of norepinephrine at the receptor. More recent studies indicate that various tricyclic antidepressants act at the cell membrane to inhibit entry of norepinephrine into the neuron.[144]

After acute administration in animals, desmethylimipramine and protriptyline caused a greater inhibition of norepinephrine-^{3}H uptake into brain than imipramine or nortriptyline.[145] Amitriptyline, in contrast, did not appear to cause an inhibition of norepinephrine uptake in brain in two studies performed in vivo,[145,146] but apparently conflicting findings have been reported.[143] The magnitude of the effects of these various tricyclic antidepressants on norepinephrine uptake are inversely correlated with their relative sedative effects after acute administration clinically — that is, amitriptyline is most sedative, whereas protriptyline and desmethylimipramine are least sedative. Since amitriptyline is metabolized to the demethylated derivative nortriptyline, which does inhibit the uptake of norepinephrine, the inhibition of monoamine uptake may be of importance in the clinical antidepressant action of amitriptyline that requires chronic drug administration. Desmethylimipramine has been suggested as the active demethylated metabolite of imipramine,[97] but contrary to earlier reports, desmethylimipramine has not proved to be a more potent or more rapidly acting antidepressant than imipramine. Tricyclic antidepressants do not appear to inhibit the uptake of dopamine into dopamine-containing neurons in the brain.[147,148]

In animals, tricyclic antidepressants also alter the metabolism of norepinephrine in the brain. Tritiated norepinephrine (norepinephrine-^{3}H) injected into the ventricular system or basal cisterns mixes with endogenous norepinephrine and appears to be a valid tracer for this amine;[149,150] the effects of drugs on norepinephrine metabolism in brain have been studied with this technic. After treatment with a number of tricyclic antidepressants, including imipramine, desmethylimipramine, protriptyline, nortriptyline and amitriptyline, levels of tritiated normetanephrine in brain are increased and tritiated deaminated catechol metabolites are decreased.[145,148,151] In clinical studies of depressed patients, decreased urinary excretion of 3-methoxy-4-hydroxymandelic acid (VMA),* the major deaminated O-methylated metabolite of norepinephrine in man, has been observed with imipramine as well as with phenelzine (a monoamine oxidase inhibitor).[125,152] These findings suggest that these tricyclic antidepressants or their metabolites prevent the deamination of norepinephrine by mitochondrial monoamine oxidase.

There is some evidence from studies in vitro that tricyclic antidepressants in high concentration may inhibit monoamine oxidase,[153,154] which could account for these findings, but other possibilities must be considered. Tricyclic antidepressants may act at intraneuronal membranes (for example, mitochondrial membranes) to prevent norepinephrine from interacting with monoamine oxidase,[125] but this has not been directly demonstrated. It is possible, therefore, that tricyclic antidepressants may exert actions at various neuronal membranes — presynaptic or postsynaptic, as well as intraneuronal — and that the effect of any given drug may depend upon the relative potencies of action at these various membrane sites.[155,156] For example, whereas the potentiation of norepinephrine produced by moderate doses of tricyclic antidepressants may result from the inhibition of inactivation by presynaptic neuronal uptake of norepineph-

* Most urinary VMA, however, probably derives from norepinephrine coming from the peripheral sympathetic nervous system rather than from the brain.[81]

rine, the adrenolytic effect observed with high doses of tricyclic antidepressants may be explained by an overriding block of the postsynaptic receptor at the higher dose.

Acute administration of imipramine or desmethylimipramine in animals slows the disappearance of intracisternally administered norepinephrine-^{3}H from brain, suggesting a decrease in turnover of norepinephrine.[149,151] In apparent conflict with these findings, however, it has been reported that administration of desmethylimipramine increases the turnover of norepinephrine in brain when this is determined by the technic of synthesis inhibition.[157]

Because chronic administration of tricyclic antidepressants is required to obtain clinically observable antidepressant effects, it has been of interest to examine the effects of chronically administered drugs on norepinephrine-^{3}H metabolism in brain. In recent experiments, after chronic administration of imipramine twice daily for three weeks, the uptake of intracisternally administered norepinephrine-^{3}H in brain was inhibited, while levels of normetanephrine-^{3}H were increased and tritiated deaminated catechol metabolites were decreased. These changes are similar to those seen after acute administration. In contrast to the findings observed after acute administration of imipramine, however, the disappearance of norepinephrine-^{3}H from brain was not slowed after chronic administration of this drug. Moreover, after chronic administration of imipramine, levels of endogenous norepinephrine in brain were lower than control values, whereas levels of endogenous norepinephrine in brain were not altered by acute administration of imipramine.[157a,157b] These differences between the effects of acutely and chronically administered imipramine on norepinephrine turnover and metabolism may provide clues to explain the need for chronic administration of this drug in the treatment of depressions.

The characteristic behavioral syndrome (that is, sedation) does not occur when reserpine is administered to animals previously treated with tricyclic antidepressants; such animals instead show an increase in behavioral activity.[158] This excitation may result from a spillover of free catecholamines onto receptors, since excitation is not observed with this combination of drugs if catecholamines are previously depleted by α-methylmetatyrosine. Deamination of norepinephrine released by reserpine is relatively decreased after pretreatment with desmethylimipramine, and free extraneuronal norepinephrine and normetanephrine are relatively increased.[159] Although these observations are compatible with the hypothesis that the excitation produced by reserpine in animals treated with desmethylimipramine depends upon the release of norepinephrine onto receptors, they may only reflect the decrease in deamination of norepinephrine generally seen with tricyclic antidepressants.[145]

As noted, tricyclic antidepressants enhance many of the peripheral effects of serotonin, although certain actions of serotonin are blocked by large doses of these drugs.[14,137] Until very recently, many investigators questioned whether the tricyclic antidepressants inhibit the uptake of serotonin in brain, and such statements are frequently seen in the literature. Studies in vitro, however, support the idea that certain tricyclic antidepressants may inhibit serotonin uptake in brain, although this has not been consistently observed in studies in vivo. When studied in vitro, both imipramine and desmethylimipramine inhibit the uptake of serotonin into brain slices[89,90] and isolated nerve endings.[160–162] In contrast, imipramine, but not desmethylimipramine, inhibited the uptake of serotonin into brain in vivo after this amine was injected into the lateral ventricle.[163,164] The uptake of radioactive serotonin in the brain also was not inhibited by desmethylimipramine in a study in which the ventricles were perfused with this amine.[165] In another study neither imipramine nor desmethylimipramine decreased the uptake of intracisternally administered radioactive serotonin in the brain.[166]

Many factors may account for these discrepant findings. Since higher concentrations of serotonin were generally used in studies performed in vivo than in the studies done in vitro, it is possible that effects of tricyclic antidepressants on specific transport mechanisms were masked by the entry of serotonin into the brain by nonspecific diffusion. Serotonin administered by intraventricular injection may be bound at sites different from those containing the endogenously formed serotonin.[167] Differences in drug doses, schedules of injection and routes of administration, or differences in regions of brain examined in the various studies, may also have contributed to the discrepancies in findings. The possibility of differences in the uptake and metabolism of serotonin in vivo and in vitro must also be considered.

Imipramine has been reported to slow the disappearance of endogenous serotonin from the brains of animals after serotonin synthesis was interrupted with α-propyldopacetamide, a tryptophan hydroxylase inhibitor; this effect was not observed with desmethylimipramine.[168,169] Similarly, imipramine, but not desmethylimipramine, slowed the disappearance of intracisternally administered radioactive serotonin from the brain.[166] These findings suggest that imipramine may decrease the turnover of serotonin in the brain.

Studies of the effects of tricyclic antidepressants on the metabolism of serotonin in brain are difficult to interpret. Levels of the deaminated metabolite, 5-hydroxyindoleacetic acid (5HIAA), formed from endogenous serotonin have been reported to be decreased by imipramine.[170] Neither imipramine nor desmethylimipramine, however, produced clear-cut changes in the levels of deaminated metabolites formed from intracisternally administered radioactive serotonin in the brain.[166] In a study in which radioactive serotonin was perfused through the lateral ventricle of rats, desmethylimipramine was found to decrease levels of endogenous but not radioactive 5HIAA in brain.[165] Moreover, desmethylimipramine did appear to slow the release from brain of radioactive 5HIAA that had been administered by intraventricular injection.[171] In clinical studies, decreased urinary excretion of 5HIAA has been observed after treatment with imipramine, but only a small fraction of urinary 5HIAA is thought to derive from the brain.[172]

Amphetamine

The acute stimulant and euphoriant effects of amphetamine in man are well established,[173] but this drug is of little value in the treatment of the major depressive disorders. Amphetamine inhibits the neuronal uptake of norepinephrine in brain; increased levels of normetanephrine-^{3}H and decreased levels of tritiated deaminated catechol metabolites are found in brain after intraventricular injection of norepinephrine-^{3}H.[147,148,174,175] Amphetamine also appears to release norepinephrine and dopamine from neurons.[148,176] Because of these and similar findings, it has been suggested that amphetamine might exert its central effects indirectly by releasing catecholamines and preventing the inactivation of these monoamines at central adrenergic synapses in the brain. However, amphetamine also decreases the uptake of serotonin into brain slices.[90]

Amphetamine counteracts the effects of reserpine in man as well as in animals.[177] The finding that amphetamine could still produce psychomotor stimulation after biogenic amines are depleted by reserpine has been interpreted by some to indicate that amphetamine might exert a direct action at various receptors in brain.[178–180] On the other hand, at least some aspects of the psychomotor stimulation produced by amphetamine in animals appear to depend upon the presence of catecholamines in the brain, particularly newly synthesized catecholamines.[119,181–184] When the synthesis of catecholamines is inhibited by α-methylparatyrosine, administration of amphetamine does not produce the usual stimulation of activity in animals.[119,182,184] The actions of amphetamine are restored after administration of the precursor of dopamine and norepinephrine, dopa, which is formed under normal physiologic conditions by the enzymatic hydroxylation of tyrosine (that is, by tyrosine hydroxylase).[181] In apparent contradiction to these findings, however, amphetamine, under certain conditions, has been reported to counteract behavioral depression produced by α-methylparatyrosine.[185] Differences in drug doses or schedules of administration or in the behavioral responses under study may account for these discrepancies. Inhibition of serotonin synthesis with parachlorophenylalanine does not appear to decrease the behavioral stimulation produced by amphetamine.[184]

Large doses of amphetamine lower the concentration of brain norepinephrine in animals[180,186–188] but cause small elevations in serotonin levels.[187] Tachyphylaxis occurs clinically with amphetamine, and the acute psychomotor stimulation, particularly after large doses, is often followed by a "rebound" depression and fatigue.[173] These changes may reflect a temporary depletion of catecholamines available for continued release.

Imipramine is known to potentiate many of the behavioral effects of amphetamine,[183,189-191] but the mechanism is not clear. Imipramine possibly potentiates the effects of norepinephrine released by amphetamine, but since imipramine slows the metabolic inactivation of amphetamine, a more direct mechanism for the observed potentiation may exist.[192,193]

Cocaine

Cocaine, a stimulant and euphoriant,[35] potentiates the effects of norepinephrine and serotonin in many physiologic systems.[194] The neuronal uptake of norepinephrine in brain appears to be inhibited by cocaine in vitro and in vivo.[174,195] Increased levels of normetanephrine-^{3}H and decreased tritiated deaminated catechol metabolites of intracisternally administered norepinephrine-^{3}H are found in the brains of animals previously treated with cocaine.[195] This drug also inhibits serotonin uptake in brain slices and isolated synaptosomes in vitro.[89,90,160]

Electroconvulsive Shock

Electroconvulsive shock remains the most effective treatment for some severely depressed patients. Examination of the effects of electroconvulsive shock on biogenic amine metabolism in animals show that levels of norepinephrine in brain decrease after repeated electroconvulsive shock.[196,197] However, levels of serotonin increase,[198-200] but not all authors concur.[201] Similar changes in norepinephrine and serotonin levels have been observed in brain after various forms of prolonged stress.[202,203] After electroconvulsive shock, altered levels of serotonin, norepinephrine or dopamine were found in one or another region of the brain. Similar (but smaller) changes, however, were also observed in "pseudoshocked" animals, and the "stress" of the shock situation may contribute to the changes seen after electroconvulsion.[204]

When norepinephrine-^{3}H is injected intracisternally before electroconvulsive shock, levels of norepinephrine-^{3}H in brain are decreased (in relation to control values) in shocked animals. Normetanephrine-^{3}H levels, however, are concurrently increased. Hence, the rate of neuronal discharge of norepinephrine onto receptors in brain may be increased by electroconvulsive shock.[195] Moreover, it has been observed that repeated electroconvulsive shock induces a sustained increase in the synthesis and utilization of norepinephrine in brain, which might account for the sustained therapeutic effects of electroconvulsive shock.[205] A similar increase in the turnover of norepinephrine in the brain, however, has been found in animals after repeated electrical shocks to the feet.[206]

Higher levels of dopamine and its deaminated O-methylated metabolite, homovanillic acid, have been found in rat brain after electroconvulsive shock.[207] After chronic administration of electroconvulsive shock to dogs, levels of 5-hydroxyindoleacetic acid as well as homovanillic acid were increased in the cerebrospinal fluid.[208] These findings indicate that electroconvulsive shock may increase the turnover of dopamine and serotonin in brain.

Lithium Salts

The effectiveness of lithium salts in the treatment of mania stimulated interest in the study of the effects of lithium on norepinephrine and serotonin metabolism. Lithium chloride has been found to cause an absolute or relative increase in levels of tritiated deaminated metabolites of intracisternally administered norepinephrine-^{3}H in rat brain and a small decrease in levels of normetanephrine-^{3}H.[209,210] Lithium salts may thus increase the deamination of norepinephrine in the brain and decrease the norepinephrine available to receptors. Corresponding to these findings in animals, urinary excretion of VMA, the major deaminated O-methylated metabolite of norepinephrine in man, was increased, whereas urinary excretion of normetanephrine and metanephrine was reduced in one study of patients treated with lithium salts.[211]

Lithium salts also appear to increase the turnover of norepinephrine in brain, as evidenced by greater depletion of norepinephrine from brain after inhibition of norepinephrine synthesis[212,213] and by an increase in the rate of disappearance of intracisternally administered norepinephrine-^{3}H from brain.[210,214] The uptake of norepinephrine-^{3}H into synaptosomes isolated from rat brain has been reported to be increased after chronic administration of lithium carbonate.[215] The uptake of intracisternally administered norepinephrine-^{3}H into rat brain (in vivo), however, was not significantly changed after the acute administration of lithium chloride,[151] nor was a statistically significant change in norepinephrine-^{3}H uptake into brain (in vivo) seen after chronic treatment with lithium chloride.[210]

The disappearance of serotonin from rat brain after inhibition of the synthesis of this amine was not found to be significantly altered after acute administration of lithium salts.[212] In contrast, lithium salts have been observed to slow the disappearance of intracisternally administered radioactive serotonin from brain and to raise levels of radioactive deaminated metabolites.[166] Since lithium salts may alter the transport of acids in kidney and brain,[216] changes in clearance from brain may account, in part, for the increases in deaminated metabolites of intracisternally administered radioactive serotonin and norepinephrine found in the brain after treatment with lithium salts.

Summary of Neuropharmacologic Studies

The effects of drugs or electroconvulsive shock on the metabolism of biogenic amines in the brain of the experimental animal seem to correlate with the effects of these treatments on affective states in man. Norepinephrine is the monoamine which has been studied most extensively, and the findings from these studies provide the most coherent body of data.

Antidepressants such as the monoamine oxidase inhibitors or the tricyclic compounds, stimulants such as cocaine or amphetamine and electroconvulsive shock all cause changes in the metabolism of norepinephrine which suggest an increase of norepinephrine at central noradrenergic receptors. In contrast, reserpine-like drugs, which can produce clinical depressions, or lithium salts, which are effective in the treatment of manias, may decrease the norepinephrine available to receptors in the brain (Table 2). These findings suggest that some, if not all, depressions may be associated with a relative deficiency of norepinephrine or other catecholamines at functionally important adrenergic receptor sites in the brain, whereas manias may be associated with an excess of catecholamines. This is known as the catecholamine hypothesis of affective disorders.[15]

It must be stressed that this formulation is not to be taken as a restrictive hypothesis, since there is also some correlation between the clinical effects of various treatments used in the affective disorders and the effects of

TABLE 2. *Summary of Effects of Psychoactive Drugs and Electroconvulsive Shock on Norepinephrine Metabolism and Mood*

Drug or Treatment	Effects on Mood (Man)	Effects on Norepinephrine Metabolism in Brain (Animals)	Presumed Effect on Norepinephrine at Receptors
Monoamine oxidase inhibitors	Antidepressant	Inhibits deamination; increases NE; increases NMN; decreases DCM	Increase
Tricyclic antidepressants	Antidepressant	Inhibits cellular uptake of NE; increases NMN; decreases DCM	Increase
Amitriptyline		May not inhibit cellular uptake of NE but increases NMN; decreases DCM	
Cocaine	Stimulant	Inhibits cellular uptake of NE; increases NMN; decreases DCM	Increase
Amphetamine	Stimulant	Inhibits cellular uptake of NE; discharges NE; increases NMN; decreases DCM	Increase
Electroconvulsive shock	Counteracts depression	Increases neuronal discharge of NE; increases NMN	Increase
Reserpine	Causes depression	Depletes NE (with intracellular deamination); decreases synthesis of NE	Decrease
Lithium salts	Counteracts mania	Increases DCM; decreases NMN; high dose increases turnover of NE	Decrease

KEY: NE = norepinephrine; NMN = normetanephrine; DCM = deaminated catechol metabolites.
SOURCE: Modified from Schildkraut, Schanberg, Breese and Kopin, *Am. J. Psychiat.* 124:600–608, 1967.

these treatments on the metabolism of the indoleamine serotonin. Correlations alone, however, cannot establish causal connections, and it cannot be determined from these data whether the alterations in monoamine metabolism necessarily cause or even contribute to the clinical effects of these drugs on mood in man. Moreover, since many of the biochemical changes may be observed in animals after acute administration of these drugs, further investigation will be required to explain the need for chronic administration of these agents (e.g., monoamine oxidase inhibitors, tricyclic antidepressants, lithium salts) in order to obtain clinical effects in the treatment of depressions and manias.

4

EXPERIMENTAL CLINICAL PHARMACOLOGY

A number of drugs or drug combinations have been used experimentally either in the treatment of affective disorders or in studies that examined their effects on mood in human subjects. These various modalities of treatment are yet to be fully evaluated either for efficacy or for safety. None of these procedures can be regarded as standard treatment regimens at present, and in some cases the occurrence of dangerous side effects strongly contraindicates routine clinical application. These experimental regimens are considered here because of their theoretical interest, irrespective of their possible clinical applications.

The amino acid precursors of the catecholamines and indoleamines can cross the blood-brain barrier, and these agents have been administered to depressed patients, as well as to other human subjects, to study effects on mood. Tryptophan, the indoleamine precursor, was the only one of several amino acids that produced mood elevation in patients with chronic schizophrenia when administered in conjunction with a monoamine oxidase inhibitor;[217] tryptophan given alone to normal subjects produces various clinical signs and symptoms, including euphoria and drowsiness.[218] In depressed patients, the therapeutic effects of monoamine oxidase inhibitors are potentiated by tryptophan, and even without the addition of monoamine oxidase inhibitors, tryptophan may be effective in the treatment of depressions.[219-221] The antidepressant activity of monoamine oxidase inhibitors may also be potentiated by 5-hydroxytryptophan in some patients,[222,223] but this effect has not been observed by all investigators.[224] The alterations in mood produced by these amino acid precursors of indoleamines need not necessarily result from an increase in indoleamines at receptors in brain, however, since these substances may also release norepinephrine centrally.[108]

Dopa, a precursor of catecholamines, was ineffective in the treatment of depression in two studies.[224,225] Since peripherally administered dopa does not readily penetrate into the parenchyma of the brain in animals,[117] it cannot be assumed that levels of catecholamines in brain were increased by the administration of dopa at the doses used in these clinical studies, particularly after oral administration. The very large doses of dopa that are required in the treatment of parkinsonism[226] raise further questions concerning the adequacy of the amounts of orally administered dopa that have been given to depressed patients. In other studies, elevation of mood has been reported in a group of patients treated with a monoamine oxidase inhibitor and dopa,[227] and improvement in depressed patients has been observed after intravenous administration of this amino acid.[228,229] Dopa may produce severe hypertension and cardiac arrhythmias when administered with a monoamine oxidase inhibitor.[230]

Tricyclic antidepressants have been used in combination with a number of other pharmacologic agents in the experimental treatment of depressed patients. Clinical improvement has been observed when reserpine or tetrabenazine has been added to the therapeutic regimen of a small number of depressed patients who have failed to respond to tricyclic antidepressants alone.[231-233] This seems to correspond to the observation that reserpine-like agents produce excitement in animals previously treated with imipramine; in animals this phenomenon has been found to depend upon the release of catecholamines.[158] In the clinical situation, however, the degree of improvement appears to correlate with the increase of 5-hydroxyindoleacetic acid excretion after reserpine, but this could be only a nonspecific indicator of the pharmacologic activity of reserpine.[233]

Tricyclic antidepressants when administered in combination with monoamine oxidase inhibitors may be effective in the treatment of some patients who fail to respond to one or another of these agents administered singly. Serious side effects can occur with this combination of drugs, however, and the combined administration of tricyclic antidepressants and monoamine oxidase inhibitors is generally considered to be too dangerous for routine clinical use.[2,5]

In a recent study, small doses of triiodothyronine, when combined with usual therapeutic doses of imipramine, produced more rapid improvement in retarded depressed patients than imipramine alone.[234] The investigators have suggested that triiodothyronine may be exerting its clinical effect by enhancing the sensitivity of adrenergic receptors to norepinephrine. Compatible with this hypothesis is the observation that thyroidectomized rats have an increased synthesis and discharge of norepinephrine that may be a compensatory response to decreased noradrenergic receptor sensitivity in hypothyroidism.[235] The greater sensitivity to norepinephrine observed in hyperthyroid patients[236] is also compatible with this hypothesis.

Two groups of investigators have recently reported that methysergide, a serotonin antagonist, may be effective in the treatment of mania.[237,238] The studies, however, were not double-blind trials, and replication under such conditions is needed. These findings would be compatible with a disturbance of indoleamine metabolism in manic states, and one of the investigators has proposed that methysergide may exert its clinical effect in mania by antagonizing "tryptamine receptors" in brain.[239,240]

Alpha-methylparatyrosine, which blocks the synthesis of catecholamines, has been administered to hypertensive patients. In these clinical trials (in which only partial inhibition of catecholamine synthesis has been attained) "sedation" is often observed when this drug is first administered. Some patients have become depressed during treatment with α-methylparatyrosine; these patients tend to have prior histories of depressive disorders. Transient hypomanic-like reactions frequently occur upon withdrawal of α-methylparatyrosine.[241,242] After administration of parachlorophenylalanine, the inhibitor of serotonin synthesis, to patients with carcinoid syndrome, psychotic confusional states, sometimes with a depressive component, have been observed in some patients.[243]

5

BIOGENIC AMINE METABOLISM IN PATIENTS WITH AFFECTIVE DISORDERS

THE effects of psychoactive drugs on the metabolism of biogenic amines have prompted studies of biogenic amine metabolism in patients with affective disorders. Direct biochemical assay of brain tissue in living man is, of course, not feasible. Most research has therefore involved assay of the monoamines or their metabolites in one or another body fluid. Various aspects of this literature have been reviewed.[11,15,16,28,244–247]

Catecholamines

In a number of studies of manic-depressive patients, the urinary excretion of norepinephrine and epinephrine has been found to be relatively lower during periods of depression than during periods of mania[248–249a] or after recovery.[250] In a large series of manic patients, excretion of both norepinephrine and epinephrine was elevated above control values, but catecholamine excretion in a heterogeneous group of depressed patients was not different from control values; depressed patients, however, did have a lowered catecholamine response to insulin stress.[251] Increased catecholamine excretion has been observed in some depressed patients,[252] but mainly in those with agitated or anxious depressions.[246,253] Depressed patients with delusions or hallucinations have been found to excrete higher levels of catecholamines and metabolites than patients who did not manifest these psychotic symptoms.[152,254]

A gradual rise in the excretion of normetanephrine — the metabolite that may reflect noradrenergic activity[71,72] — occurred during the period of definitive clinical improvement in a series of patients with endogenous depressions treated with imipramine.[51] In this longitudinal study, patients with retarded depressions had lower levels of normetanephrine excretion before treatment (when depressed) than after clinical remission.[51] In contrast, some patients with agitated depressions were found to have higher levels of normetanephrine, as well as norepinephrine and epinephrine, when depressed than after improvement.[253] Normetanephrine and metanephrine excretion has been reported to be elevated in association with agitated, unstable behavior in depressed patients and in others.[255] After infusion with radioactive norepinephrine, patients with retarded depressions, classified as manic depressions, were found to have an elevated ratio of radioactive amines to deaminated metabolites in the urine;[256] many factors, including an alteration in the disposition of infused norepinephrine, could account for these findings. Increased excretion of catecholamines and metabolites, including normetanephrine, has been observed in manic and hypomanic patients, and the magnitudes of the normetanephrine elevations were related to the clinical severity of the hypomanic symptoms.[51,257]

Since not all studies have employed a uniform system for classifying the depressions, it is difficult to compare the findings. In general, however, norepinephrine and normetanephrine excretion appears to be decreased in patients with retarded (endogenous) depressions and increased in patients with mania. The findings in patients with agitated or anxious depressions are less consistent, and some of these patients seem to show increased excretion of norepinephrine and normetanephrine as well as epinephrine and metanephrine.

The interpretation of these findings must be made with the awareness that factors other than emotional state — for example, muscular activity — may produce significant changes in urinary norepinephrine excretion.[258] Moreover, because of the relatively effective blood-brain barrier to norepinephrine and normetanephrine,[82,259-261] it is probable that only a small fraction of urinary norepinephrine or normetanephrine derives from the brain. Thus, urinary excretion of norepinephrine and normetanephrine primarily reflects the activity of the peripheral sympathetic nervous system.

The sulfate conjugate of 3-methoxy-4-hydroxyphenylglycol (MHPG), an O-methylated deaminated metabolite of norepinephrine, is the major metabolite of normetanephrine in rat brain.[82] Most norepinephrine coming from brain is excreted in the urine as MHPG in dogs.[81] Although technical difficulties have prevented comparable studies of these routes of metabolism of norepinephrine in human brain, the sulfate conjugate of MHPG has been found in the cerebrospinal fluid of man.[262] The urinary excretion of MHPG, therefore, may provide a more direct index of central noradrenergic activity in man than any of the other metabolites of norepinephrine, although urinary MHPG may also derive, in part, from norepinephrine coming from peripheral sympathetic nerves.

Urinary MHPG excretion was significantly lower in a diagnostically heterogeneous group of depressed patients than in a nondepressed control population.[263] In a small group of depressed patients studied longitudinally, levels of urinary MHPG were consistently lower during the depression than after clinical remission; these values were also considerably lower than MHPG levels observed in any of the other patients in this study.[253] Hypomanic patients, in contrast, had higher levels of MHPG excretion before clinical remission.[253] These findings are thus compatible with but do not definitively establish the hypothesis that a decrease in central noradrenergic activity may occur in at least some depressions, whereas central noradrenergic activity may be increased in manias.[15]

Indoleamines

The urinary excretion of 5-hydroxyindoleacetic acid (5HIAA) in patients with affective disorders has been studied extensively.[224,244,247,248,264–267] In some of these studies excretion of 5HIAA was decreased in patients with agitated depressions and increased in those with retarded depressions; manic patients also had increased 5HIAA excretion. However, since it is thought that much urinary 5HIAA may derive from indoleamines in the gastrointestinal tract,[264,268] and that dietary factors may be of considerable importance, relatively little may be inferred from such observations about the metabolism of serotonin in the central nervous system.

Studies in animals suggest that more direct information concerning serotonin metabolism in the brain may be obtained from studies of 5HIAA in cerebrospinal fluid.[269] Decreased levels of 5-hydroxyindoles (principally 5HIAA) in cerebrospinal fluid have been reported in depressed patients, with normal values observed upon recovery.[270,271] Levels of 5-hydroxyindoles in hypomanic or manic patients have been reported to be decreased[271] or normal.[270] Since a concentration gradient of 5HIAA appears to exist within the cerebrospinal fluid system, and exercise may affect values obtained after lumbar punctures,[270,272] further studies will be required to establish the meaning of these findings.

In a postmortem study of depressed patients after suicide, levels of serotonin in the hind brain were lower than in the control group.[273] This observation, however, was not replicated in a more recent study, but 5HIAA was reported to be lower in depressed patients after suicide than in control subjects after death from natural causes; statistically significant differences in levels of norepinephrine were not observed.[274] As the investigators pointed out, interpretation of these very provocative data is exceedingly difficult because of the many uncontrolled variables that may have influenced the result of these studies. Included among these are the ingestion of psychoactive drugs before the suicide, the age differences between the suicide and control groups and, perhaps most importantly, the fact that many of the low values of 5HIAA observed in the patients after suicide seemed to be associated with barbiturate ingestion.

Urinary tryptamine excretion is decreased in depressed patients and returns to normal levels after clinical improvement;[264,275] the import of this observation, however, is not clear. Depressed patients had a relatively decreased rate of liberation of $^{14}CO_2$ from carboxy-labeled 5-hydroxytryptophan in one study,[276] but the group originally reporting this finding did not observe the phenomenon in a further study of depressed patients.[245] Most urinary tryptamine probably derives from the decarboxylation of tryptophan in the kidney, and relatively little may be of central origin; dietary factors may also cause alterations in tryptamine excretion.[264,275] Excretion of xanthurenic acid, a product of the major (kynurenine) pathway of tryptophan metabolism, may be greater in depressed than in manic patients.[277] Thus, a shift in the pathways of metabolism of tryptophan, leading to a decreased synthesis of indoleamines, may account in part both for the decrease in tryptamine excretion as well as for some of the other changes in indoleamine metabolism which have been reported to occur in depressive disorders.[278–280]

6

DIFFERENTIAL DIAGNOSIS AND TREATMENT OF DEPRESSIVE DISORDERS

THIS chapter provides a brief outline of the criteria which I use for the differential diagnosis of the depressive disorders, as well as suggestions for their treatment. It must be reemphasized, however, that an appreciable number of patients will fall within the ill-defined areas separating one or another of the diagnostic categories and will not be classified uniquely according to the system presented. Moreover, as with any nosological system based only on clinical signs and symptoms, the possibility of misdiagnosis must always be considered. The suggestions for treatment, therefore, are offered only as recommendations for the initial trial of therapy. If improvement does not occur after a suitable therapeutic trial of one treatment approach, the physician may be advised to try alternative measures. Since depressions constitute a recurrent problem for many patients, clues to successful therapy may be found in the history of previous responses to one or another form of treatment. If a particular treatment has proved successful in previous episodes, the likelihood of its future success is enhanced. All patients with depressive disorders, irrespective of diagnostic type, may be suicidal. The risk of suicide, therefore, must be recognized and evaluated in every depressed patient. These factors must temper the recommendations provided in the following outline.

Endogenous Depressions

Endogenous depressions, which account for no more than 10 to 20 per cent of all depressive disorders, include:

1. Manic-depressive depressions
2. Recurrent depressions
3. Nonrecurrent depressions
4. Involutional depressions

Endogenous depressions are characterized by psychic retardation; decrease in interest and ambition; loss of initiative; impaired sense of vitality; the inability to anticipate or attain the usual satisfactions or pleasures customarily obtained from work or recreational activities; and associated feelings of hopelessness, helplessness, worthlessness and guilt. Sadness of affect (i.e., depression as a symptom) is often but not invariably present. In the endogenous depressions, the depressive syndrome is generally reported to be qualitatively different from those depressions of mood which the patient has experienced during the normal course of everyday life. Endogenous depressions are further characterized by the autonomy of the depressive syndrome once it has been established (irrespective of whether or not the depression was initially precipitated by events in the patient's life) and by the lack of reactivity of the symptoms either to alterations in the patient's environment or to social or therapeutic interpersonal interactions. Diurnal variation in the intensity of symptoms, typically a worsening in the morning and partial remission later in the day, is often noted. Other commonly occurring symptoms include sleep disturbance (typically with early morning awakening) and anorexia (sometimes with appreciable weight loss). Patients with endogenous depressions usually present histories of adequate premorbid social adjustment and a previous capacity to function well at work. Recovery from episodes of endogenous depressions usually occurs with complete clinical remission. Thus the depressive episodes in such patients can be fairly well separated from both the premorbid and postmorbid intervals.

Several subgroups have been suggested within the group of endogenous depressions. Manic-depressive depressions are identified by a history of at least one prior well-documented manic or hypomanic episode. Recurrent depressions may be indistinguishable clinically from manic-depressive depressions except for the absence of a history of manic episodes. Some recurrent depressions may, indeed, be variants of manic-depressive alternations, and the appearance of a manic episode after many episodes of recurrent depressions is not uncommon. The nonrecurrent depressions are distinguished from the former two subgroups by the absence of a prior history of mania or depression. Such a depression may, of course, represent the first episode in either a manic-depressive or a recurrent depression, but some patients may have only one episode in a lifetime. The involutional depressions are clinically distinguished by the presence of greater motor agitation (e.g., hand-wringing and pacing), feelings or delusions of guilt, somatic preoccupations which are frequently delusional, and paranoid ideation and delusions. While the other endogenous depressions may occur for the first time in the late teens or at any age thereafter, the diagnosis of involutional depression can rarely, if ever, be made in a patient under the age of 35, and involutional depressions most commonly occur only after the age of 45.

An initial trial of treatment with a tricyclic antidepressant is usually warranted in patients with endogenous depressions. Because of the delay in onset of the therapeutic effects of tricyclic antidepressants, however, electroconvulsive therapy may be the preferred form of treatment for some patients with endogenous depressions, particularly those judged to be highly suicidal. Phenothiazines may be useful in the treatment of involutional depressions in which agitation and paranoid delusions are prominent symptoms. Electroconvulsive therapy, however, remains the most strikingly effective form of treatment for the involutional depressions.

Schizoaffective Depressions

The schizoaffective depressions are those depressions which occur in the context of a schizophrenic, schizoid or borderline illness.[20,29] The primary treatment of a schizoaffective depression should be directed toward the underlying schizophrenic or borderline disorder. Antipsychotic drugs such as phenothiazines are often useful in the treatment of patients with schizoaffective disorders. The tricyclic antidepressants may also be of some value, but these agents, like the monoamine oxidase inhibitors, may precipitate overt psychotic episodes in such patients.

Chronic Characterologic Depressions

The chronic characterologic depressions are seen in those patients whose depressions are an inherent part of a life-long personality problem in which relatively minor stresses or changes in life patterns may precipitate symptomatology. Such patients characteristically show poor premorbid adjustments, but the term *premorbid* usually has little real meaning in this group. These patients typically present symptoms such as unhappiness, dissatisfaction, helplessness, dependency, demandingness, a sense of entitlement, irritability, anger, emotional lability and histrionic behavior.

Patients with chronic characterologic depressions often show transient improvement with all forms of therapeutic intervention, including supportive interpersonal therapy or simply hospitalization; but sustained definitive clinical improvement is rare. Intensive psychotherapy is generally indicated for the long-term treatment of patients with chronic characterologic depressions. Although most of these patients are not particularly responsive to treatment with the major antidepressant drugs, some patients fitting this clinical description do appear to improve during treatment with one of the major antidepressants. A therapeutic trial of a tricyclic antidepressant or a monoamine oxidase inhibitor, therefore, may be indicated if initial psychotherapeutic intervention does not achieve a remission of the symptoms in a patient with a chronic characterologic depression.

Situational Depressions

The situational depressions (sometimes called "reactive" depressions) are those depressive disorders which occur as a result of an overwhelming situational stress. These depressions are very common and include the depressive states of pathologic grief and mourning. Situational depressions are self-limited disorders, and remission usually occurs within a few months. Supportive psychotherapy is generally the treatment of choice. Occasionally a situational depression may evolve into what appears to be an endogenous depressive disorder in which the symptoms become autonomous of the initial precipitating stress or the subsequent related life events. Under such conditions, treatment of the disorder should proceed as with any other endogenous depression.

Neurochemical and Clinical Speculations on the Treatment of Endogenous Depressions

The neuropharmacologic and clinical neurochemical findings reviewed above suggest the possibility that a neurochemical lesion (e.g., decreased monoamine synthesis, increased monoamine inactivation or decreased receptor sensitivity) within noradrenergic or other monoaminergic neuronal systems may occur in cases of endogenous depressions; this could result in a functional deficiency of norepinephrine or other monoamines at critical receptor sites in the brain. In contrast, it has been speculated that the other depressive disorders (i.e., the schizoaffective, chronic characterologic and situational depressions) may be associated with various abnormalities of input into monoaminergic neuronal systems, either from the environment or from various centers in the brain; these may secondarily result in a decrease in the activity of one or another monoaminergic neuronal system without a primary neurochemical abnormality within monoaminergic neurons per se. If this admittedly speculative formulation is valid, in endogenous depressions the repair of the underlying neurochemical lesion within the monoaminergic neuronal systems, either by antidepressant drugs or electroconvulsive therapy, would seem necessary before other therapeutic approaches, for example, psychotherapy or environmental manipulation, could be expected to be effective.

The initial phase of treatment of endogenous depressions, in fact, consists of the administration of antidepressant drugs (or electroconvulsive therapy when this is considered to be the treatment of choice — see above). A period of one to four weeks generally elapses from the time of initial administration of tricyclic antidepressants to the onset of definitive clinical improvement.

Although the patient may appear to be relatively unresponsive to interpersonal interactions during this phase of treatment, a great deal of important interpersonal work nonetheless can occur as the physician offers support and optimism. Moreover, it is essential to provide the patient with a realistic assessment of his prognosis (which is very good in cases of endogenous depressions) in order to counter his depressive sense of hopelessness and despair. The goals of the therapeutic work during this phase are to build a firm, trusting relationship with the patient and to keep him from acting on his suicidal wishes. Attempts to mobilize the patient into purposeful activity at this stage are often unsuccessful and may only reinforce the patient's sense of inadequacy. Support of the patient's realistic attempts to maintain his activities during this period is important, however, in order to prevent a further loss of self-esteem. Excessive expectations for performance (whether coming from the patient or from the physician) should be avoided, since these may result in failure which will further decrease the patient's already impaired sense of self-esteem and increase his feelings of worthlessness.

When a patient with an endogenous depression starts to improve on antidepressant drugs, the effect is often striking. The exact day of onset of clinical improvement can generally be defined, and the psychiatrist can usually ascertain this upon visual inspection. The patient's carriage may appear to be more erect, his movements may be less restricted and more agile and his face may be more expressive. The patient characteristically becomes more responsive to environmental stimuli at this time, and during this phase of the treatment of patients with endogenous depressions it may be of value to attempt to activate the patient through the use of various interpersonal techniques in order to promote both affective arousal and the resumption of purposeful activity. Timing is of critical importance here, as the physician must be certain that the patient is no longer suicidal before attempting to do this. Confrontation over relevant issues and the attendant mobilization of affect, including anger, which often occur at this stage in the treatment of such patients, may serve an important function beyond that of simple exploration of the content of the issues involved. Implicit in this approach is the notion that noradrenergic or other monoaminergic neuronal systems may be operative both in the normal regulation of affective states and levels of arousal as well as in the maintenance of a sense of initiative and a capacity to execute active coping behavior.[11] Moreover, it is suggested that these affective states and behavioral responses (e.g., affective arousal and active coping behavior), which may at first be initiated by the activity of monoaminergic neurons, may, under normal conditions, then serve to increase the activity of these neuronal systems* by a positive feedback mechanism. This hypothesized positive feedback could account for the well-known clinical examples of the depressed patient whose depression seems to perpetuate further depression and the manic patient whose elation and hyperactivity lead to further escalation of the mania.

It is generally recognized that decreasing environmental stimulation serves an important function in the management of the manic patient. The reversal of this technique, moreover, may be of use in the treatment of the patient with an endogenous depression once clinical improvement has begun. Increasing the environmental input to promote affective arousal and a sense of initiative, as well as purposeful action and active coping be-

* A means of regulating (i.e., setting limits on) such a system would of course be required to prevent its unlimited escalation.

havior, may lead to a progressively self-perpetuating improvement in affective state in such patients recovering from endogenous depressions. Thus the effective (and socially appropriate) expression of aggression may be of considerable importance, whereas the antidepressant drugs, which may have been necessary to achieve an initial neuropharmacologic pump-priming action (i.e., the initial activation of monoaminergic neuronal systems), may be of less importance during this phase of the treatment of patients with endogenous depressions. It has been our experience in treating patients with active milieu therapy on a research ward that some patients with endogenous depressions may be withdrawn from tricyclic antidepressant medication immediately after the onset of clinical improvement without exacerbation of the depression.[51,152] Clinical conservatism, however, would suggest a more gradual schedule of withdrawal of antidepressant drugs (as outlined below) in routine practice.

After complete clinical remission has been attained, the dose of antidepressant medication often may be reduced to a lower maintenance level. I generally recommend that this be done very gradually (e.g., imipramine or amitriptyline may be decreased by 25 milligrams every seven to fourteen days). When the appropriate maintenance dose level is reached, administration of the drug is generally continued for at least several months at this reduced dose. In those patients for whom long-term maintenance therapy is not contemplated, the eventual discontinuation of the drug should proceed gradually. (Here, too, I suggest that the dose of imipramine or amitriptyline be decreased by 25 milligrams every seven to fourteen days.) The physician must observe his patient carefully and often during this period, and he should be prepared to increase the drug dosage if the symptoms of depression recur.

APPENDIXES

Appendix I

APPROXIMATE DAILY DOSE RANGES OF THE MAJOR ANTIDEPRESSANT DRUGS

THE approximate dose ranges listed in Table A-1 are intended only as general guidelines for therapy. When prescribing any of these antidepressants, the physician must be familiar with the pharmacology of the particular drug and must accordingly take into account the specific clinical characteristics of the individual patient, including his response to the drug. It is usually advisable to start medication at a fairly low dose and to increase it gradually over a number of days in order to attain a therapeutically effective dose. Similarly, when one of these antidepressants is to be discontinued electively, it is advisable to withdraw the drug gradually. Withdrawal symptoms may occur upon abrupt cessation of some antidepressants. The doses required for maintenance therapy with specific tricyclic or monoamine oxidase inhibitor antidepressants may fall below even the lower limits of the dose ranges suggested in Table A-1 for active antidepressant treatment. Elderly patients generally tolerate these drugs less well, and lower doses are usually recommended for them. Because of the opportunity for closer clinical observation and the greater restriction of activities of patients in the hospital, the maximum doses which may be administered to hospitalized patients sometimes exceed the maximum doses recommended by the pharmaceutical company for outpatients. Thus, for some of the antidepressants, the upper limits of the dose ranges outlined in Table A-1 may not necessarily be recommended for the treatment of outpatients.

TABLE A-1. *Approximate Daily Dose Ranges of Major Antidepressant Drugs*

Generic Name	Brand Name	Approximate Dose Range (Mg/Day)
	TRICYCLIC ANTIDEPRESSANTS	
Imipramine	Tofrānil	100–200 (up to 300)
Amitriptyline	Elavil	100–150 (up to 300)
Desipramine	Pertofrane, Norpramin	100–200
Nortriptyline	Aventyl	40–100
Protriptyline	Vivactil	30–60
	MONOAMINE OXIDASE INHIBITORS	
Phenelzine	Nardil	45–75
Tranylcypromine	Parnate	20–30
Nialamide	Niamid	75–200
Isocarboxazid	Marplan	20–30

Appendix II

CONTRAINDICATIONS, PRECAUTIONS AND SIDE EFFECTS ASSOCIATED WITH THE USE OF THE MAJOR ANTIDEPRESSANT DRUGS

THIS appendix outlines the more common and many of the less common contraindications, precautions and side effects associated with the use of the two major classes of antidepressant drugs. While this outline is rather broadly inclusive, it cannot be assumed to be exhaustive. The physician must, therefore, be alert to the possibility that a patient may present contraindications to the use of these drugs or side effects induced by these drugs which are not included in this outline. It must also be noted that each of the relative contraindications or precautions associated with a particular class of antidepressants need not necessarily apply to every drug within that class. Moreover, it must be stressed that each of the side effects ascribed to one or the other class of major antidepressants has not necessarily been observed with all of the drugs within that class.

No attempt has been made to document the relative frequency of the various side effects listed, since the reliability of such information, where it is available, is often problematic. In clinical practice, it is frequently difficult to be certain that a particular adverse effect has necessarily been caused by administration of a particular drug. This is especially a problem with the antidepressants, since many of the commonly observed side effects are also symptoms which are associated with depressive syndromes per se, e.g., dry mouth and constipation.

In the present outline, side effects have been organized according to the major physiologic or organ system involved. Where it was felt that interests of clarity would be served best by classifying a particular side effect under more than one system, this has been done. Discussion of the possible physiologic mechanisms underlying these side effects or their possible treatments was not considered to be within the scope of this appendix, which is intended to serve only as a summary outline and a brief clinical guide.

Tricyclic Antidepressants

CONTRAINDICATIONS OR REASONS FOR PRECAUTION

- Medical conditions
  - Cardiovascular disease
  - Glaucoma — increased intraocular pressure
  - Urine retention
  - Prostatic hypertrophy
  - Pyloric stenosis
  - Hyperthyroidism
  - Epilepsy
  - Schizophrenia
  - Liver disease
  - Pregnancy or childbearing potential
  - Lactation
  - Children under age 12
  - Prior history of hypersensitivity to the specific tricyclic antidepressant under consideration
- Pharmacologic agents
  - Monoamine oxidase inhibitors
  - Anticholinergic agents
  - Sympathomimetic drugs

- Antihypertensive agents, particularly guanethidine
- Thyroid medications
- Alcohol

SIDE EFFECTS

- Autonomic nervous system effects (mainly anticholinergic)
  - Postural hypotension
  - Tachycardia
  - Sweating, particularly over head, neck and shoulders
  - Flushing
  - Dry mouth
  - Impaired visual accommodation
  - Blurred vision
  - Mydriasis
  - Aggravation of glaucoma
  - Constipation
  - Paralytic ileus
  - Urinary bladder atonia
  - Urine retention
- Other nervous system effects
  - Tremor
  - Dizziness
  - Headache
  - Sense of pressure or fullness in ears or head
  - Tinnitus
  - Drowsiness*
  - Insomnia*
  - Weakness
  - Incoordination
  - Ataxia
  - Vertigo
  - Fainting
  - Paresthesias

* Amitriptyline is more sedative than imipramine, whereas protriptyline has minimal sedative effects.

- Peripheral neuropathy
- Dysarthria
- EEG changes
- Seizures
- Parkinson-like syndrome
- Dystonia

Psychiatric effects

- Anxiety and jitteriness
- Hypomanic or manic episodes
- Activation of psychosis in schizophrenic patients
- Hostility
- Nightmares
- Confusional states
- Visual hallucinations

Cardiovascular and renal effects

- Hypotension
- Hypertension
- Tachycardia
- Palpitations
- ECG changes, including flattened T waves, depressed S-T segments, prolonged Q-T intervals, prolonged conduction time
- Myocardial infarction
- Congestive heart failure
- Edema
- Urinary frequency
- Nocturia

Oral, gastrointestinal and hepatic effects

- Dry mouth (and secondary oral and dental problems)
- Bad taste
- Black tongue
- Sublingual adenitis
- Increased appetite and weight gain
- Heartburn
- Anorexia

- Nausea
- Vomiting
- Abdominal pain
- Diarrhea
- Altered liver function tests
- Jaundice (obstructive)
- Constipation
- Paralytic ileus

Sexual effects
- Increase or decrease in libido
- Impotence

Metabolic and endocrine effects
- Increased appetite and weight gain
- Gynecomastia
- Galactorrhea

Allergic and hypersensitivity reactions
- Skin rash
- Urticaria
- Itching
- Photosensitivity
- Petechiae
- Eosinophilia
- Swelling of face and tongue

Hematologic effects
- Bone marrow depression
- Leukopenia
- Agranulocytosis
- Thrombocytopenia
- Purpura

Monoamine Oxidase Inhibitor Antidepressants

CONTRAINDICATIONS OR REASONS FOR PRECAUTION

Medical conditions
- Cardiovascular disease, including hypertension and hypotension
- Pheochromocytoma

- Cerebrovascular defects
- Headaches (or history of headaches)
- Epilepsy
- Schizophrenia
- Hyperthyroidism
- Liver disease or altered liver function tests
- Kidney disease or impairment of renal function
- Pregnancy or childbearing potential
- Lactation
- Debilitation
- Old age (over age 60)
- Elective surgery
- General or spinal anesthesia

Pharmacologic agents

- Tricyclic antidepressants
- Other monoamine oxidase inhibitors
- Sympathomimetic drugs, including stimulants, diet pills and vasoconstrictors
- Dopa or methyldopa
- Norepinephrine, epinephrine or dopamine
- Tryptophan
- Cocaine or procaine
- Narcotics, particularly meperidine
- Sedatives and hypnotics, including barbiturates and chloral hydrate
- Alcohol
- Antihypertensive agents
- Diuretics
- Caffeine
- Hypoglycemic agents
- Antihistaminics
- Antiparkinsonism drugs
- Anesthetics
- Antimalarials
- Reserpine or reserpine-like drugs

Foods containing monoamines, sympathomimetic amines or their precursors, e.g., tyramine or dopa

Dietary substances implicated in hypertensive crises*

- Cheeses, particularly aged varieties
- Wines, particularly Chianti
- Beer
- Alcohol
- Pickled herring
- Broad bean pods (fava beans)
- Chicken liver
- Yeast extract
- Snails
- Caffeine

SIDE EFFECTS

Autonomic nervous system effects

- Postural hypotension
- Tachycardia
- Sweating
- Dry mouth
- Blurred vision
- Glaucoma
- Constipation

Other nervous system effects

- Dizziness
- Weakness and fatigue
- Drowsiness
- Insomnia
- Anxiety
- Jitteriness
- Akathisia
- Tremors
- Muscle twitching

* This list contains the most commonly cited substances; it cannot be considered complete, however, as other foods may also cause hypertensive crises in patients treated with monoamine oxidase inhibitors.

- Hyperreflexia
- Seizures
- Headache (may indicate hypertensive crisis — see below)
- Ataxia
- Nystagmus
- Toxic delirium
- Coma
- Anorexia
- Peripheral neuropathy

Psychiatric effects

- Anxiety and jitteriness
- Euphoria
- Hypomania and mania
- Activation of psychosis in schizophrenic patients

Cardiovascular and renal effects

- Hypotension
- Tachycardia
- Palpitations
- Hypertension and hypertensive crises*
- Suppression of anginal pain
- Edema
- Hypernatremia
- Delayed micturition
- Urine retention

Gastrointestinal and hepatic effects

- Anorexia
- Nausea
- Constipation
- Diarrhea

* Hypertensive crises are characterized by some or all of the following signs and symptoms: headache (usually occipital which may radiate frontally); neck stiffness or soreness; palpitations; tachycardia or bradycardia; chest pain; vomiting; sweating; fever; cold, clammy skin; photophobia; dilated pupils. Intracranial bleeding may occur. Deaths have been reported.

- Jaundice (hepatocellular)
- Necrotizing hepatocellular damage

Sexual effects
- Disturbances in sexual functions
- Impotence
- Delayed ejaculation

Metabolic and endocrine effects
- Possible potentiation of hypoglycemic agents

Allergic and hypersensitivity reactions
- Skin rash
- Photosensitivity
- Edema of glottis

Hematologic effects
- Anemia
- Leukopenia
- Agranulocytosis

Other effects
- Transient respiratory and cardiovascular depression after electroconvulsive therapy

Appendix III

CHEMICAL FORMULAS OF THE MAJOR ANTIDEPRESSANT DRUGS AND RELATED COMPOUNDS

THIS appendix provides the chemical formulas of the major antidepressant drugs as well as a number of other drugs which have been used in the treatment of the affective disorders. The formulas of the biogenic amines have also been included so that they may be compared with the various psychoactive drugs depicted.

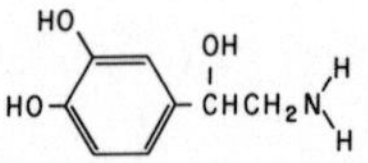

NOREPINEPHRINE

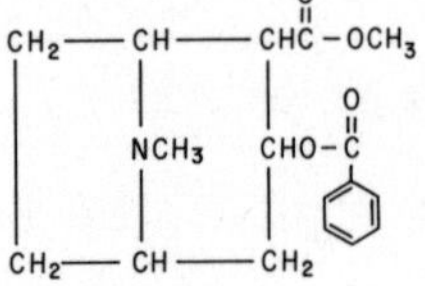

COCAINE

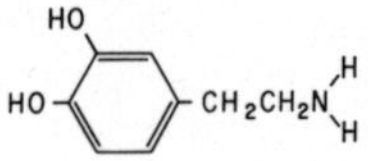

DOPAMINE

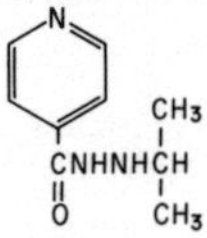

IPRONIAZID

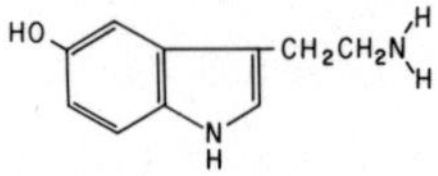

SEROTONIN

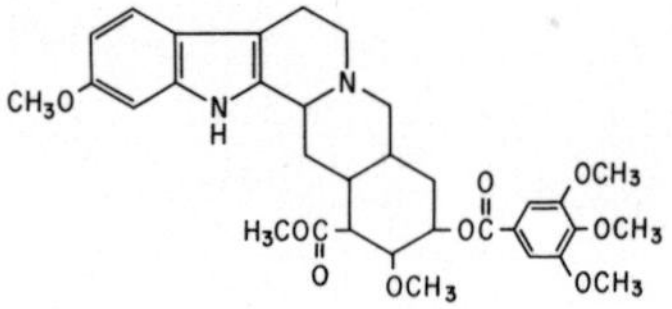

RESERPINE

FIGURE A-1. *Compounds of Theoretical or Historical Interest.*

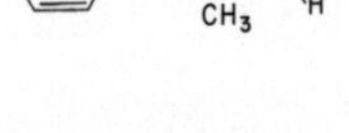

AMPHETAMINE

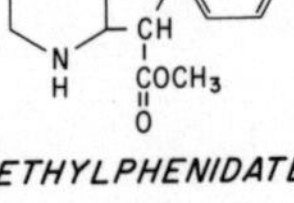

METHYLPHENIDATE

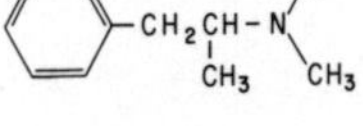

METHAMPHETAMINE

FIGURE A-2. *Stimulants and Euphoriants.*

Chemical Formulas of the Antidepressant Drugs

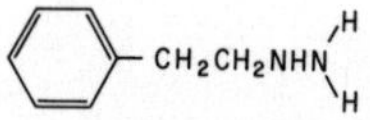

PHENELZINE

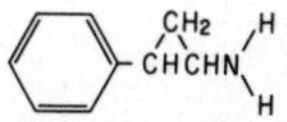

TRANYLCYPROMINE

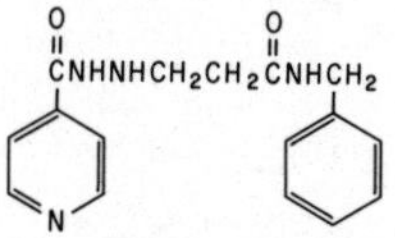

NIALAMIDE

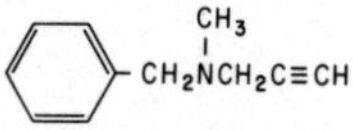

PARGYLINE

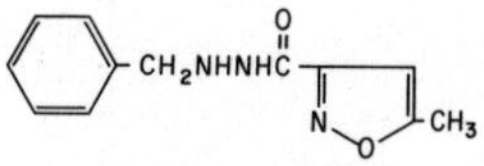

ISOCARBOXAZID

FIGURE A-3. *Monoamine Oxidase Inhibitors.*

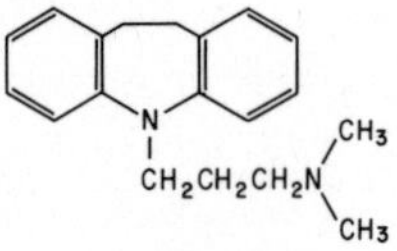

IMIPRAMINE

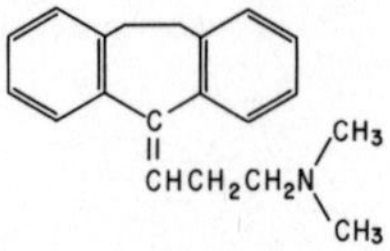

AMITRIPTYLINE

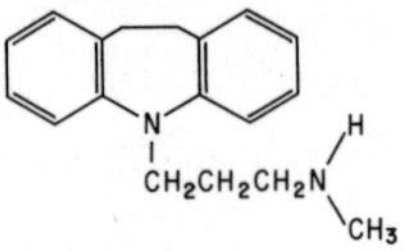

DESIPRAMINE
DESMETHYLIMIPRAMINE

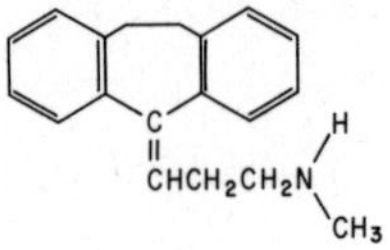

NORTRIPTYLINE
DESMETHYLAMITRIPTYLINE

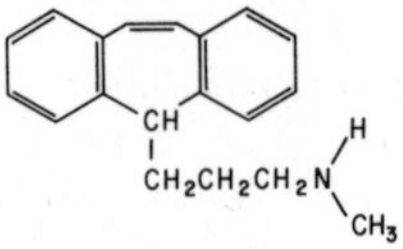

PROTRIPTYLINE

FIGURE A-4. *Tricyclic Antidepressants.*

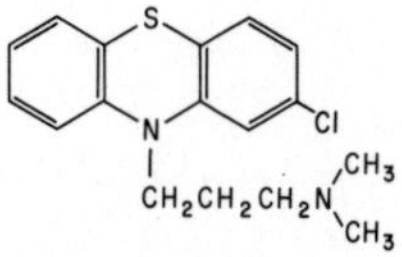

CHLORPROMAZINE
(Phenothiazine Derivative)

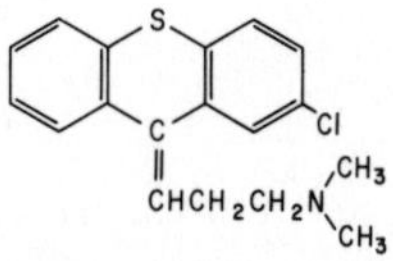

CHLORPROTHIXENE
(Thioxanthene Derivative)

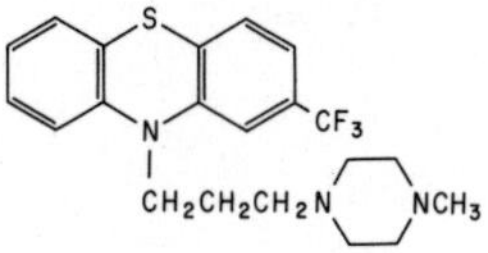

TRIFLUOPERAZINE
(Phenothiazine Derivative)

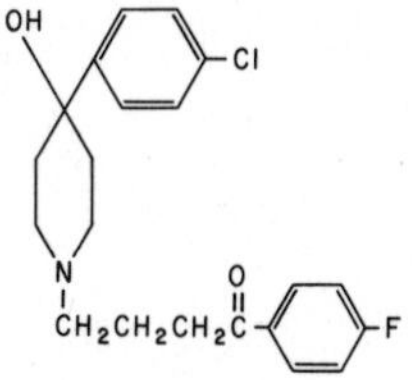

HALOPERIDOL
(Butyrophenone Derivative)

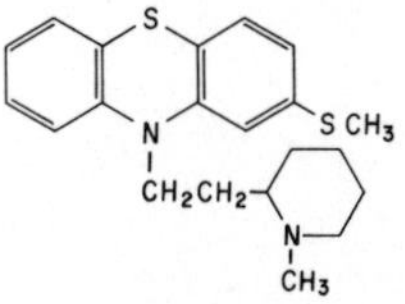

THIORIDAZINE
(Phenothiazine Derivative)

FIGURE A-5. *Prototypic Antipsychotic Agents Used in Affective Disorders.*

REFERENCES

REFERENCES

1. Davis, J. M., Klerman, G. L., and Schildkraut, J. J. Drugs used in treatment of depressions. In United States Department of Health, Education, and Welfare, Public Health Service. *Psychopharmacology, Review of Progress, 1957–67: Proceedings of the 6th annual meeting of the American College of Neuropsychopharmacology, San Juan, Puerto Rico, December 12–15, 1967*. Editor-in-chief D. H. Efron. Washington, D.C.: U.S. Government Printing Office, 1968. (Publication No. 1836.) Pp. 719–747.
2. Shepherd, M., Lader, M., and Rodnight, R. *Clinical Psychopharmacology*. London: English Universities Press, 1968.

2a. Klein, D. F., and Davis, J. M. *Diagnosis and Drug Treatment of Psychiatric Disorders*. Baltimore: Williams & Wilkins, 1969.

3. Schou, M. Lithium in psychiatric therapy and prophylaxis. *J. Psychiat. Research* 6:67–95, 1968.
4. Lehmann, H. E. Clinical perspectives on antidepressant therapy. *Am. J. Psychiat.* (Suppl.) 124:12–21, May, 1968.
5. Cole, J. O., and Davis, J. M. Antidepressant drugs. In *Comprehensive Textbook of Psychiatry*. Edited by A. M. Freedman and H. I. Kaplan. Baltimore: Williams & Wilkins, 1967. Pp. 1263–1275.
6. Klerman, G. L., and Cole, J. O. Clinical pharmacology of imipramine and related antidepressant compounds. *Pharmacol. Rev.* 17: 101–141, 1965.
7. Hordern, A. Antidepressant drugs. *New Eng. J. Med.* 272:1159–1169, 1965.
8. Bloom, F. E., and Giarman, N. J. Physiologic and pharmacologic considerations of biogenic amines in nervous system. *Ann. Rev. Pharmacol.* 8:229–258, 1968.
9. Glowinski, J., and Baldessarini, R. J. Metabolism of norepinephrine in central nervous system. *Pharmacol. Rev.* 18:1201–1238, 1966.
10. Wurtman, R. J. *Catecholamines*. Boston: Little, Brown, 1966.
11. Schildkraut, J. J., and Kety, S. S. Biogenic amines and emotion. *Science* 156:21–30, 1967.
12. Freedman, D. X. Aspects of biochemical pharmacology of psychotropic drugs. In *Psychiatric Drugs*. Edited by P. Solomon. New York: Grune & Stratton, 1966. Pp. 32–57.

13. Pletscher, A. Monoamine oxidase inhibitors: Effects related to psychostimulation. In United States Department of Health, Education, and Welfare, Public Health Service. *Psychopharmacology, Review of Progress, 1957–67: Proceedings of the 6th annual meeting of the American College of Neuropsychopharmacology, San Juan, Puerto Rico, December 12–15, 1967.* Editor-in-chief D. H. Efron. Washington, D.C.: U.S. Government Printing Office, 1968. (Publication No. 1836.) Pp. 649–654.
14. Sigg, E. B. Tricyclic thymoleptic agents and some newer antidepressants. In United States Department of Health, Education, and Welfare, Public Health Service. *Psychopharmacology, Review of Progress, 1957–67: Proceedings of the 6th annual meeting of the American College of Neuropsychopharmacology, San Juan, Puerto Rico, December 12–15, 1967.* Editor-in-chief D. H. Efron. Washington, D.C.: U.S. Government Printing Office, 1968. (Publication No. 1836.) Pp. 655–669.
15. Schildkraut, J. J. Catecholamine hypothesis of affective disorders: Review of supporting evidence. *Am. J. Psychiat.* 122:509–522, 1965.
16. Bunney, W. E., Jr., and Davis, J. M. Norepinephrine in depressive reactions: Review. *Arch. Gen. Psychiat.* 13:483–494, 1965.
17. Durell, J., and Schildkraut, J. J. Biochemical studies of schizophrenic and affective disorders. In *American Handbook of Psychiatry,* Vol. III. Edited by S. Arieti. New York: Basic Books, 1966. Pp. 423–457.
17a. Kraepelin, E. *Manic-Depressive Insanity and Paranoia.* Edinburgh: Livingstone, 1921.
18. Lewis, A. J. Melancholia: Historical review. *J. Ment. Sc.* 80:1–42, 1934.
19. Kendell, R. E. *The Classification of Depressive Illnesses.* London: Oxford University Press, 1968. (No. 18, *Institute of Psychiatry, Maudsley Monographs.*)
20. Ewalt, J. R., and Farnsworth, D. L. *Textbook of Psychiatry.* New York: McGraw-Hill, 1963.
21. Hamilton, M., and White, J. M. Clinical syndromes in depressive states. *J. Ment. Sc.* 105:985–998, 1959.
22. Mendelson, M. *Psychoanalytic Concepts of Depression.* Springfield, Illinois: Thomas, 1960.
23. Grinker, R. R., Miller, J., Sabshin, M., Nunn, R., and Nunnally, J. C. *The Phenomena of Depressions.* New York: Harper, 1961.
24. Friedman, A. S., Cowitz, B., Cohen, H. W., and Granick, S. Syndromes and themes of psychotic depression: Factor analysis. *Arch. Gen. Psychiat.* 9:504–509, 1963.
25. Kiloh, L. G., and Garside, R. F. Independence of neurotic depression and endogenous depression. *Brit. J. Psychiat.* 109:451–463, 1963.
26. Beck, A. T. *Depression: Clinical, Experimental, and Theoretical Aspects.* New York: Harper & Row, 1967.
27. Mendels, J., and Cochrane, C. Nosology of depression: Endogenous-reactive concept. *Am. J. Psychiat.* (Suppl.) 124:1–11, May, 1968.
28. Schildkraut, J. J., Davis, J. M., and Klerman, G. L. Biochemistry

of depressions. In United States Department of Health, Education, and Welfare, Public Health Service. *Psychopharmacology, Review of Progress, 1957–67: Proceedings of the 6th annual meeting of the American College of Neuropsychopharmacology, San Juan, Puerto Rico, December 12–15, 1967.* Editor-in-chief D. H. Efron. Washington, D.C.: U.S. Government Printing Office, 1968. (Publication No. 1836.) Pp. 625–648.

29. American Psychiatric Association, Committee on Nomenclature and Statistics. *Diagnostic and Statistical Manual of Mental Disorders.* Second edition. Washington, D.C.: American Psychiatric Association, 1968.
30. Rosenthal, S. H., and Klerman, G. L. Content and consistency in endogenous depressive pattern. *Brit. J. Psychiat.* 112:471–484, 1966.
31. Rosenthal, S. H. Involutional depressive syndrome. *Am. J. Psychiat.* (Suppl.) 124:21–35, May, 1968.
32. Winokur, G., and Clayton, P. Family history studies. I. Two types of affective disorders separated according to genetic and clinical factors. *Recent Advances in Biol. Psychiat.* 9:35–50, 1967.
33. Perris, C. Study of bipolar (manic-depressive) and unipolar recurrent depressive psychoses. *Acta psychiat. Scandinav.* (Suppl.) 194(42): 7–188, 1966.
34. Angst, J. Zur Ätiologie und Nosologie endogener depressiver Psychosen: Eine genetische, soziologische und klinische Studie. *Monogr. Neurol. Psychiat.* 112:1–118, 1966.
35. Freud, S. *The Cocaine Papers.* Vienna: Dunquin, 1963.
36. Myerson, A. Effect of benzedrine sulfate on mood and fatigue in normal and in neurotic persons. *Arch. Neurol. & Psychiat.* 36:816–822, 1936.
37. Peoples, S. A., and Guttmann, E. Hypertension produced with benzedrine: Its psychological accompaniments. *Lancet* 1:1107–1109, 1936.
38. Crane, G. E. Iproniazid (Marsilid) phosphate, therapeutic agent for mental disorders and debilitating diseases. *Psychiat. Research Rep.* 8:142–152, 1957.
39. Loomer, H. P., Saunders, J. C., and Kline, N. S. Clinical and pharmacodynamic evaluation of iproniazid as psychic energizer. *Psychiat. Research Rep.* 8:129–141, 1957.
40. Kuhn, R. Treatment of depressive states with G 22355 (imipramine hydrochloride). *Am. J. Psychiat.* 115:459–464, 1958.
41. Greenblatt, M., Grosser, G. H., and Wechsler, H. Differential response of hospitalized depressed patients to somatic therapy. *Am. J. Psychiat.* 120:935–943, 1964.
42. Innes, I. R., and Nickerson, M. Drugs acting on postganglionic adrenergic nerve endings and structures innervated by them (sympathomimetic drugs). In *The Pharmacological Basis of Therapeutics.* Third edition. Edited by L. S. Goodman and A. Gilman. New York: Macmillan, 1965. Pp. 477–520.
43. Weiss, B., and Laties, V. G. Enhancement of human performance by caffeine and amphetamines. *Pharmacol. Rev.* 14:1–36, 1962.

44. Roberts, J. M. Prognostic factors in electroshock treatment of depressive states. I. Clinical features from history and examination. *J. Ment. Sc.* 105:693–702, 1959. Prognostic factors in electroshock treatment of depressive states. II. Application of specific tests. *Ibid.* 105:703–713, 1959.
45. Fawcett, J. A., Siomupoulos, V., and Maas, J. W. Personal communication, 1969.
46. Zeller, E. A., and Barsky, J. *In vivo* inhibition of liver and brain monoamine oxidase by 1-isonicotinyl-2-isopropyl hydrazine. *Proc. Soc. Exper. Biol. & Med.* 81:459–461, 1952.
47. West, E. D., and Dally, P. J. Effects of iproniazid in depressive syndromes. *Brit. M. J.* 1:1491–1494, 1959.
48. Pare, C. M. B., Rees, L., and Sainsbury, M. J. Differentiation of two genetically specific types of depression by response to antidepressants. *Lancet* 2:1340–1343, 1962.
49. Kiloh, L. G., Ball, J. R. B., and Garside, R. F. Prognostic factors in treatment of depressive states with imipramine. *Brit. M. J.* 1: 1225–1227, 1962.
50. Raskin, A. Prediction of antidepressant drug effects: Review and critique. In United States Department of Health, Education, and Welfare, Public Health Service. *Psychopharmacology, Review of Progress, 1957–67: Proceedings of the 6th annual meeting of the American College of Neuropsychopharmacology, San Juan, Puerto Rico, December 12–15, 1967.* Editor-in-chief D. H. Efron. Washington, D.C.: U.S. Government Printing Office, 1968. (Publication No. 1836.) Pp. 757–765.
51. Schildkraut, J. J., Green, R., Gordon, E. K., and Durell, J. Normetanephrine excretion and affective state in depressed patients treated with imipramine. *Am. J. Psychiat.* 123:690–700, 1966.
52. Fink, M., Klein, D. F., and Kramer, J. C. Clinical efficacy of chlorpromazine-procyclidine combination, imipramine and placebo in depressive disorders. *Psychopharmacologia* 7:27–36, 1965.
53. Hollister, L. E., and Overall, J. E. Phenothiazine derivatives as antidepressants. *Agressologie* 4:289–292, 1968.
54. Paykel, E. S., Price, J. S., Gillan, R. U., Palmai, G., and Chesser, E. S. Comparative trial of imipramine and chlorpromazine in depressed patients. *Brit. J. Psychiat.* 114:1281–1287, 1968.
55. Raskin, A. High dosage chlorpromazine alone and in combination with antiparkinsonian agent (procyclidine) in treatment of hospitalized depressions. *J. Nerv. & Ment. Dis.* 147:184–195, 1968.
56. Cade, J. F. J. Lithium salts in treatment of psychotic excitement. *M. J. Australia* 2:349–352, 1949.
57. Baastrup, P. C., and Schou, M. Lithium as prophylactic agent: Its effect against recurrent depressions and manic-depression psychosis. *Arch. Gen. Psychiat.* 16:162–172, 1967.
58. Blackwell, B., and Shepherd, M. Prophylactic lithium: Another therapeutic myth? Examination of evidence to date. *Lancet* 1:968–971, 1968.
59. Fieve, R. R., Platman, S. R., and Plutchik, R. R. Use of lithium in

affective disorders. I. Acute endogenous depression. *Am. J. Psychiat.* 125:487–491, 1968. Use of lithium in affective disorders. II. Prophylaxis of depression of chronic recurrent affective disorders. *Ibid.* 125:492–498, 1968.
60. Vogt, M. Concentration of sympathin in different parts of central nervous system under normal conditions and after administration of drugs. *J. Physiol.* 123:451–481, 1954.
61. von Euler, U. S. *Noradrenaline: Chemistry, Physiology, Pharmacology and Clinical Aspects.* Edited by R. F. Pitts. Springfield, Illinois: Thomas, 1956. (No. 261, *American Lecture Series, Monograph in Bannerstone Division of American Lectures in Physiology.*)
62. Vogt, M. Catecholamines in brain. *Pharmacol. Rev.* 11:483–489, 1959.
63. Carlsson, A., Lindqvist, M., and Magnusson, T. On biochemistry and possible functions of dopamine and noradrenaline in brain. In Ciba Foundation, *Adrenergic Mechanisms (Papers and Discussions)*, Editor for British Pharmacological Society: J. R. Vane. Editors for Foundation: G. E. W. Wolstenholme and M. O'Connor. Boston: Little, Brown, 1961. (*Symposia, General Series.*) Pp. 432–439.
64. Crawford, T. B. B. Distribution of 5-hydroxytryptamine in central nervous system of dog. In Symposium on 5-Hydroxytryptamine. *5-Hydroxytryptamine: Proceedings of a Symposium Held in London on 1st-2d April 1957.* Edited by G. P. Lewis. New York: Pergamon, 1958. Pp. 20–25.
65. Crossland, J. Role of monoamines in excitation and depression of central nervous system. In Symposium on the Clinical Chemistry of Monoamines, Manchester, England, 1962. *The Clinical Chemistry of Monoamines (Proceedings): Organized by the Association of Clinical Biochemists.* Edited by H. Varley and A. H. Gowenlock. Amsterdam: Elsevier, 1963. (Vol. 2. *West European Symposia on Clinical Chemistry.*) Pp. 175–190.
66. McLennan, H. *Synaptic Transmission.* Philadelphia: Saunders, 1963.
67. Falck, B. Cellular localization of monoamines. In Symposium on Binding Sites of Brain Biogenic Amines, Galesburg, Illinois, 1963. *Biogenic Amines.* Edited by H. E. Himwich and W. A. Himwich. Amsterdam: Elsevier, 1964. Pp. 28–44.
68. Hillarp, N. A., Fuxe, K., and Dahlstrom, A. Demonstration and mapping of central neurons containing dopamine, noradrenaline and 5-hydroxytryptamine and their reactions to psychopharmaca. *Pharmacol. Rev.* 18:727–741, 1966.
69. Brodie, B. B., and Shore, P. A. Concept for role of serotonin and norepinephrine as chemical mediators in brain. *Ann. New York Acad. Sc.* 66:631–642, 1957.
70. Giarman, N. J. Neurohumors in brain. *Yale J. Biol. & Med.* 32:73–92, 1959.
71. Kopin, I. J., and Gordon, E. K. Metabolism of norepinephrine-H^3 released by tyramine and reserpine. *J. Pharmacol. & Exper. Therap.* 138:351–359, 1962.

72. *Idem.* Metabolism of administered and drug-released norepinephrine-7-H^3 in rat. *J. Pharmacol. & Exper. Therap.* 140:207–216, 1963.
73. Potter, L. T., and Axelrod, J. Studies on storage of norepinephrine and effect of drugs. *J. Pharmacol. & Exper. Therap.* 140:199–206, 1963.
74. Axelrod, J. Uptake and release of catecholamines and effect of drugs. In Symposium on Binding Sites of Brain Biogenic Amines, Galesburg, Illinois, 1963. *Biogenic Amines.* Edited by H. E. Himwich and W. A. Himwich. Amsterdam: Elsevier, 1964. Pp. 81–89.
75. Carlsson, A. Functional significance of drug-induced changes in brain monoamine levels. In Symposium on Binding Sites of Brain Biogenic Amines, Galesburg, Illinois, 1963. *Biogenic Amines.* Edited by H. E. Himwich and W. A. Himwich. Amsterdam: Elsevier, 1964. Pp. 9–27.
76. Costa, E., and Brodie, B. B. Concept of neurochemical transducer as organized molecular unit at sympathetic nerve endings. In Symposium on Binding Sites of Brain Biogenic Amines, Galesburg, Illinois, 1963. *Biogenic Amines.* Edited by H. E. Himwich and W. A. Himwich. Amsterdam: Elsevier, 1964. Pp. 168–185.
77. Kopin, I. J. Storage and metabolism of catecholamines: Role of monoamine-oxidase. *Pharmacol. Rev.* 16:179–191, 1964.
78. Armstrong, M. D., McMillan, A., and Shaw, K. N. F. 3-Methoxy-4-hydroxy-D-mandelic acid: Urinary metabolite of norepinephrine. *Biochim. et biophys. acta* 25:422, 1957.
79. Axelrod, J., Kopin, I. J., and Mann, J. D. 3-Methoxy-4-hydroxyphenyglycol sulfate, new metabolite of epinephrine and norepinephrine. *Biochim. et biophys. acta* 36:576, 1959.
80. Mannarino, E., Kirshner, N., and Nashold, B. S., Jr. Metabolism of (C-14) noradrenaline by cat brain *in vivo. J. Neurochem.* 10:373–379, 1963.
81. Maas, J. W., and Landis, D. H. *In vivo* studies of metabolism of norepinephrine in central nervous system. *J. Pharmacol. & Exper. Therap.* 163:147–162, 1968.
82. Schanberg, S. M., Schildkraut, J. J., Breese, G. R., and Kopin, I. J. Metabolism of normetanephrine-H^3 in rat brain — identification of conjugated 3-methoxy-4-hydroxyphenylglycol as major metabolite. *Biochem. Pharmacol.* 17:247–254, 1968.
83. Blaschko, H. Biological inactivation of 5-hydroxytryptamine. In Symposium on 5-Hydroxytryptamine. *5-Hydroxytryptamine: Proceedings of a Symposium Held in London on 1st–2d April 1957.* Edited by G. P. Lewis. New York: Pergamon, 1958. Pp. 50–57.
84. Giarman, N. J., and Schanberg, S. M. Intracellular distribution of 5-hydroxytryptamine (HT: serotonin) in rat's brain. *Biochem. Pharmacol.* 1:301–306, 1958.
85. Udenfriend, S. Metabolism of 5-hydroxytryptamine. In Symposium on 5-Hydroxytryptamine. *5-Hydroxytryptamine: Proceedings of a Symposium Held in London on 1st–2d April 1957.* Edited by G. P. Lewis. New York: Pergamon, 1958. Pp. 43–49.

86. Schanberg, S. M., and Giarman, N. J. Drug-induced alterations in sub-cellular distribution of 5-hydroxytryptamine in rat's brain. *Biochem. Pharmacol.* 11:187–194, 1962.
87. Garattini, S., and Valzelli, L. *Serotonin.* Amsterdam: Elsevier, 1965.
88. Keglević, D., Kveder, S., and Iskrić, S. Indoleacetaldehydes — intermediates in indolealkylamine metabolism. *Advances in Pharmacol.* 6:79–89, 1968.
89. Blackburn, K. J., French, P. C., and Merrills, R. J. 5-Hydroxytryptamine uptake in rat brain in vitro. *Life Sc.* 6:1653–1663, 1967.
90. Ross, S. B., and Renyi, A. L. Accumulation of tritiated 5-hydroxytryptamine in brain slices. *Life Sc.* 6:1407–1415, 1967.
91. Achor, R. W. P., Hanson, N. O., and Gifford, R. W., Jr. Hypertension treated with Rauwolfia serpentina (whole root) and with reserpine: Controlled study disclosing occasional severe depression. *J.A.M.A.* 159:841–845, 1955.
92. Muller, J. C., Pryor, W. W., Gibbons, J. E., and Orgain, E. S. Depression and anxiety occurring during Rauwolfia therapy. *J.A.M.A.* 159:836–839, 1955.
93. Lemieux, G., Davignon, A., and Genest, J. Depressive states during Rauwolfia therapy for arterial hypertension: Report of 30 cases. *Canad. M. A. J.* 74:522–526, 1956.
94. Harris, T. H. Depression induced by Rauwolfia compounds. *Am. J. Psychiat.* 113:950, 1957.
95. Ayd, F. J., Jr. Drug-induced depression: Fact or fallacy. *New York State J. Med.* 58:354–356, 1958.
96. Bernstein, S., and Kaufman, M. R. Psychological analysis of apparent depression following Rauwolfia therapy. *J. Mt. Sinai Hosp.* 27:525–530, 1960.
97. Brodie, B. B. Some ideas on mode of action of imipramine-type antidepressants. In *The Scientific Basis of Drug Therapy in Psychiatry: A Symposium at St. Bartholomew's Hospital, London, 7th–8th September 1964.* Edited by J. Marks and C. M. B. Pare. Oxford: Pergamon, 1965. Pp. 127–154.
98. Pletscher, A., Shore, P. A., and Brodie, B. B. Serotonin release as possible mechanism of reserpine action. *Science* 122:374, 1955.
99. Bertler, A., Carlsson, A., and Rosengren, E. Release by reserpine of catechol amines from rabbits' hearts. *Naturwissenschaften* 43: 521, 1956.
100. Holzbauer, M., and Vogt, M. Depression by reserpine of noradrenaline concentration in hypothalamus of cat. *J. Neurochem.* 1:8–11, 1956.
101. Shore, P. A. Release of serotonin and catecholamines by drugs. *Pharmacol. Rev.* 14:531–550, 1962.
102. Rutledge, C. O., and Weiner, N. Effect of reserpine upon synthesis of norepinephrine in isolated rabbit heart. *J. Pharmacol. & Exper. Therap.* 157:290–302, 1967.
103. Roth, R. H., and Stone, E. A. Action of reserpine on noradrenaline biosynthesis in sympathetic nerve tissue. *Biochem. Pharmacol.* 17:1581–1590, 1968.

104. Kopin, I. J., and Weise, V. K. Effect of reserpine and metaraminol on excretion of homovanillic acid and 3-methoxy-4-hydroxyphenylglycol in rat. *Biochem. Pharmacol.* 17:1461–1464, 1968.
105. Häggendal, J., and Lindqvist, M. Disclosure of labile monoamine fractions in brain and their correlation to behaviour. *Acta physiol. Scandinav.* 60:351–357, 1964.
106. Trčka, V., and Carlsson, A. Pharmacology of reserpine analogues. VI. Reserpine analogues with differential effect on brain monoamines. *Acta pharmacol. et toxicol.* 25:107–112, 1967.
107. Kety, S. S. Amino acids, amines and behavior. *Research Pub. A. Res. Nerv. & Ment. Dis.* 40:311–324, 1962.
108. Brodie, B. B., Comer, M. S., Costa, E., and Dlabac, A. Role of brain serotonin in mechanism of central action of reserpine. *J. Pharmacol. & Exper. Therap.* 152:340–349, 1966.
109. Glowinski, J., Iversen, L. L., and Axelrod, J. Storage and synthesis of norepinephrine in reserpine-treated rat brain. *J. Pharmacol. & Exper. Therap.* 151:385–399, 1966.
110. Carlsson, A., Lindqvist, M., and Magnusson, T. 3,4-Dihydroxyphenylalanine and 5-hydroxytryptophan as reserpine antagonists. *Nature* (London) 180:1200, 1957.
111. Everett, G. M., and Toman, J. E. P. Mode of action of Rauwolfia alkaloids and motor activity. In Masserman, J. H. *Biological Psychiatry*. New York: Grune, 1959. Pp. 75–81.
112. McGeer, P. L., McGeer, E. G., and Wada, J. A. Central aromatic amine levels and behavior. II. Serotonin and catecholamine levels in various cat brain areas following administration of psychoactive drugs or amine precursors. *Arch. Neurol.* 9:81–89, 1963.
113. Wada, J. A., Wrinch, J., Hill, D., McGeer, P. L., and McGeer, E. G. Central aromatic amine levels and behavior. I. Conditioned avoidance response in cats, following administration of psychoactive drugs or amine precursors. *Arch. Neurol.* 9:69–80, 1963.
114. Graeff, F. G., Leme, J. G., and Rocha e Silva, M. Role played by catechol and indolamines in central actions of reserpine after mono-aminoxidase inhibition. *Internat. J. Neuropharmacol.* 4:17–26, 1965.
115. Degkwitz, R., Frowein, R., Kulenkampff, C., and Mohs, U. Über die Wirkungen des 1-Dopa beim Menschen und deren Beeinflussung durch Reserpin, Chlorpromazin, Iproniazid und Vitamin B_6. *Klin. Wchnschr.* 38:120–123, 1960.
116. Green, H., and Sawyer, J. L. Biochemical-pharmacological studies with 5-hydroxytryptophan, precursor of serotonin. In Symposium on Binding Sites of Brain Biogenic Amines, Galesburg, Illinois, 1963. *Biogenic Amines.* Edited by H. E. Himwich and W. A. Himwich, Amsterdam: Elsevier, 1964. Pp. 150–167.
117. Bertler, A., Falck, B., Owman, C., and Rosengren, E. Localization of monoaminergic blood-brain barrier mechanisms. *Pharmacol. Rev.* 18:369–385, 1966.
118. Spector, S., Sjoerdsma, A., and Udenfriend, S. Blockade of endogenous norepinephrine synthesis by α-methyl-tyrosine, inhibitor

of tyrosine hydroxylase. *J. Pharmacol. & Exper. Therap.* 147:86–95, 1965.

119. Weissman, A., Koe, B. K., and Tenen, S. S. Antiamphetamine effects following inhibition of tyrosine hydroxylase. *J. Pharmacol. & Exper. Therap.* 151:339–352, 1966.
120. Koe, B. K., and Weissman, A. Marked depletion of brain serotonin by p-chlorophenylalanine. *Federation Proc.* 25:452, 1966.
121. Brodie, B. B., and Reid, W. D. Serotonin in brain: Functional considerations. *Advances in Pharmacol.* (Suppl.) 6B:97–113, 1968.
122. Carlsson, A. Reporter's remarks. *Advances in Pharmacol.* 6B:115–119, 1968.
123. Sjoerdsma, A., Gillespie, L., Jr., and Udenfriend, S. Simple method for measurement of monoamine-oxidase inhibition in man. *Lancet* 2:159, 1958.
124. von Studnitz, W. Effect of marsilid on excretion of 3-methoxy-4-hydroxymandelic acid in man. *Scandinav. J. Clin. & Lab. Investtigation* 11:224, 1959.
125. Schildkraut, J. J., Klerman, G. L., Hammond, R., and Friend, D. G. Excretion of 3-methoxy-4-hydroxymandelic acid (VMA) in depressed patients treated with antidepressant drugs. *J. Psychiat. Research* 2:257–266, 1964.
126. Spector, S., Shore, P. A., and Brodie, B. B. Biochemical and pharmacological effects of monoamine oxidase inhibitors, iproniazid, 1-phenyl-2-hydrazinopropane (JB 516) and 1-phenyl-3-hydrazinobutane (JB 835). *J. Pharmacol. & Exper. Therap.* 128:15–21, 1960.
127. Spector, S., Hirsch, C. W., and Brodie, B. B. Association of behavioral effects of pargyline, non-hydrazide MAO inhibitor with increase in brain norepinephrine. *Internat. J. Neuropharmacol.* 2:81–93, 1963.
128. Everett, G. M., and Wiegand, R. G. Central amines and behavioral states: Critique and new data. In International Pharmacological Meeting. *Proceedings of the First Meeting, August 22–25, 1961: Mode of Action of Drugs.* 10 vol. General editor: B. Urnäs. Vol. 8 edited by W. D. M. Paton and P. Lindgren. New York: Pergamon, 1962. Pp. 85–92.
129. Green, H., and Erickson, R. W. Further studies with tranylcypromine (monoamine oxidase inhibitor) and its interaction with reserpine in rat brain. *Arch. Internat. Pharmacodyn.* 135:407–425, 1962.
130. Corrodi, H. Blockade of psychotic syndrome caused by nialamide in mice. *J. Pharm. & Pharmacol.* 18:197–199, 1966.
131. Chessin, M., Kramer, E. R., and Scott, C. C. Modifications of pharmacology of reserpine and serotonin by iproniazid. *J. Pharmacol. & Exper. Therap.* 119:453–460, 1957.
132. Stein, L., and Ray, O. S. Accelerated recovery from reserpine depression by monoamine oxidase inhibitors. *Nature* (London) 188: 1199, 1960.
133. Carlsson, A. Brain monoamines and psychotropic drugs. In 2d International Congress of Neuro-psychopharmacology, Basle, 1960.

Proceedings. Edited by E. Rothlin. Amsterdam: Elsevier, 1961. Pp. 417–421.

134. Ryall, R. W. Effects of cocaine and antidepressant drugs on nictitating membrane of cat. *Brit. J. Pharmacol.* 17:339–357, 1961.
135. Sigg, E. B., Soffer, L., and Gyermek, L. Influence of imipramine and related psychoactive agents on effect of 5-hydroxytryptamine and catecholamines on cat nictitating membrane. *J. Pharmacol. & Exper. Therap.* 142:13–20, 1963.
136. Thoenen, H., Hürlimann, A., and Haefely, W. Mode of action of imipramine and 5-(3′-methylaminopropyliden)-dibenzo [a,e] cyclohepta [1,3,5] trien hydrochloride (Ro 4-6011), new antidepressant drug, on peripheral adrenergic mechanisms. *J. Pharmacol. & Exper. Therap.* 144:405–414, 1964.
137. Gyermek, L. Effects of imipramine-like antidepressant agents on autonomic nervous system. In *Antidepressant Drugs of Non-MAO Inhibitor Type*. Edited by D. H. Efron and S. S. Kety. Washington, D.C.: U.S. Government Printing Office, 1966. (Workshop of Pharmacology Unit, N.I.M.H., No. 1.) Pp. 41–62.
138. Gershon, S., Holmberg, G., Mattsson, E., Mattsson, N., and Marshall, A. Imipramine hydrochloride: Its effects on clinical, autonomic, and physiological functions. *Arch. Gen. Psychiat.* 6:96–101, 1962.
139. Prange, A. J., Jr., Postrom, E., and Cochrane, C. M. Imipramine enhancement of norepinephrine in normal humans. *Psychiat. Digest* 25:27–40, 1964.
140. Svedmyr, N. Influence of tricyclic antidepressive agent (protriptyline) on some of circulatory effects of noradrenaline and adrenaline in man. *Life Sc.* 7:77–84, 1968.
141. Sigg, E. B. Pharmacological studies with Tofranil. *Canad. Psychiat. A. J.* (Suppl.) 4:75–85, 1959.
142. Hertting, G., Axelrod, J., and Whitby, L. G. Effect of drugs on uptake and metabolism of H^3-norepinephrine. *J. Pharmacol. & Exper. Therap.* 134:146–153, 1961.
143. Glowinski, J., and Axelrod, J. Inhibition of uptake of tritiated-noradrenaline in intact rat brain by imipramine and related compounds. *Nature* (London) 204:1318, 1964.
144. Carlsson, A., and Waldeck, B. Mechanism of amine transport in cell membranes of adrenergic nerves. *Acta pharmacol.* 22:293–300, 1965.
145. Schildkraut, J. J., Dodge, G. A., and Logue, M. A. Effects of tricyclic antidepressants on uptake and metabolism of intracisternally administered norepinephrine-H^3 in rat brain. *J. Psychiat. Research* 7:29–34, 1969.
146. Stille, G. Pharmacological investigation of antidepressant compounds. *Pharmakopsychiatrie Neuropsychopharmakologie* 1:92–106, 1968.
147. Carlsson, A., Fuxe, K., Hamberger, B., and Lindqvist, M. Biochemical and histochemical studies on effects of imipramine-like drugs and (+)-amphetamine on central and peripheral catecholamine neurons. *Acta physiol. Scandinav.* 67:481–497, 1966.

148. Glowinski, J., Axelrod, J., and Iversen, L. L. Regional studies of catecholamines in rat brain. IV. Effects of drugs on disposition and metabolism of H^3-norepinephrine and H^3-dopamine. *J. Pharmacol. & Exper. Therap.* 153:30–41, 1966.
149. Glowinski, J., and Axelrod, J. Effects of drugs on disposition of H^3-norepinephrine in rat brain. *Pharmacol. Rev.* 18:775–785, 1966.
150. Schanberg, S. M., Schildkraut, J. J., and Kopin, I. J. Effects of pentobarbital on fate of intracisternally administered norepinephrine-H^3. *J. Pharmacol. & Exper. Therap.* 157:311–318, 1967.
151. Schanberg, S. M., Schildkraut, J. J., and Kopin, I. J. Effects of psychoactive drugs on norepinephrine-H^3 metabolism in brain. *Biochem. Pharmacol.* 16:393–399, 1967.
152. Schildkraut, J. J., Gordon, E. K., and Durell, J. Catecholamine metabolism in affective disorders. I. Normetanephrine and VMA excretion in depressed patients treated with imipramine. *J. Psychiat. Research* 3:213–228, 1965.
153. Pulver, R., Exer, B., and Herrmann, B. Einige Wirkungen des N-(γ-dimethylamino-propyl)-iminodibenzyl-HCI und seiner Metabolite auf den Stoffwechsel von Neurohormonen. *Arzneimittel-Forsch.* 10:530–533, 1960.
154. Gabay, S., and Valcourt, A. J. Biochemical determinants in evaluation of monoamine oxidase inhibitors. In Society of Biological Psychiatry. *Recent Advances in Biological Psychiatry.* Vol. 10 edited by J. Wortis. New York: Plenum, 1968. Pp. 29–41.
155. Haefely, W. Hürlimann, A., and Thoenen, H. Scheinbar paradoxe Beeinflussung von peripheren Noradrenalinwirkungen durch einige Thymoleptica. *Helvet. physiol. acta* 22:15–33, 1964.
156. Pletscher, A. Pharmacologic and biochemical basis of some somatic side effects of psychotropic drugs. In *Neuropsychopharmacology.* Edited by H. Brill et al. Amsterdam: Excerpta Medica, 1967. Pp. 571–577.
157. Neff, N. H., and Costa, E. Effect of tricyclic antidepressants and chlorpromazine on brain catecholamine synthesis. In *Anti-depressant Drugs: Proceedings. Organized by the Istituto di Ricerche Farmacologiche Mario Negri, Milan, April 25–27, 1966.* Edited by S. Garattini and M. N. G. Dukes. Amsterdam: Excerpta Medica, 1967. Pp. 28–34.
157a. Schildkraut, J. J. Changes in norepinephrine-H^3 (NE-H^3) metabolism in rat brain after acute and chronic administration of tricyclic antidepressants. *Federation Proc.* 28:795, 1969.
157b. Schildkraut, J. J., Winokur, A., and Applegate, C. W. Norepinephrine turnover and metabolism in rat brain after chronic administration of imipramine. *Science* (in press).
158. Sulser, F., Bickel, M. H., and Brodie, B. B. Action of desmethylimipramine in counteracting sedation and cholinergic effects of reserpine-like drugs. *J. Pharmacol. & Exper. Therap.* 144:321–330, 1964.
159. Sulser, F., Owens, M. L., and Dingell, J. V. *In vivo* modification of biochemical effects of reserpine by desipramine in hypothalamus of rat. *Pharmacologist* 9 (2):213, 1967.

160. Segawa, T., and Kuruma, I. Influences of drugs on uptake of 5-hydroxytryptamine by nerve-ending particles of rabbit brain stem. *J. Pharm. & Pharmacol.* 20:320–322, 1968.
161. Wise, C. D., and Ruelius, H. W. Binding of serotonin in brain: Study *in vitro* of influence of physicochemical factors and drugs. *Biochem. Pharmacol.* 17:617–631, 1968.
162. Davis, J. M., Colburn, R., Murphy, D. L., and Bunney, W. E., Jr. New research tool for study of brain biogenic amines and psychoactive drugs. In *Scientific Proceedings of the American Psychiatric Association*. Washington, D.C.: American Psychiatric Association, 1968. Pp. 228 and 229.
163. Fuxe, K., and Ungerstedt, U. Localization of 5-hydroxytryptamine uptake in rat brain after intraventricular injection. *J. Pharm. & Pharmacol.* 19:335–337, 1967.
164. Carlson, A., Fuxe, K., and Ungerstedt, U. Effect of imipramine on central 5-hydroxytryptamine neurons. *J. Pharm. & Pharmacol.* 20:150, 1968.
165. Palaić, D., Page, I. H., and Khairallah, P. A. Uptake and metabolism of (^{14}C) serotonin in rat brain. *J. Neurochem.* 14:63–69, 1967.
166. Schildkraut, J. J., Schanberg, S. M., Breese, G. R., and Kopin, I. J. Effects of psychoactive drugs on metabolism of intracisternally administered serotonin in rat brain. *Biochem. Pharmacol.* 18:1971–1978, 1969.
167. Sanders-Bush, E., and Sulser, F. Selective effect of drugs on brain serotonin at different functional "sites." *Pharmacologist* 10:210, 1968.
168. Corrodi, H., and Fuxe, K. Effect of imipramine on central monoamine neurons. *J. Pharm. & Pharmacol.* 20:230, 1968.
169. Corrodi, H., Fuxe, K., and Hökfelt, T. Effect of some psychoactive drugs on central monoamine neurons. *Europ. J. Pharmacol.* 1:363–368, 1967.
170. Da Prada, M., and Pletscher, A. On mechanism of chlorpromazine-induced changes of cerebral homovanillic acid levels. *J. Pharm. & Pharmacol.* 18:628–630, 1966.
171. Eccleston, D. Personal communication, 1968.
172. Haškovec, L., and Ryšánek, K. Excretion of 3-methoxy-4-hydroxymandelic acid and 5-hydroxyindoleacetic acid in depressed patients treated with imipramine. *J. Psychiat. Research* 5:213–220, 1967.
173. Goodman, L. S., and Gilman, A. *Pharmacological Basis of Therapeutics: A Textbook of Pharmacology, Toxicology, and Therapeutics for Physicians and Medical Students.* Second edition. New York: Macmillan, 1955. Pp. 361 and 518.
174. Dengler, H. G., Spiegel, H. E., and Titus, E. O. Effect of drugs on uptake of isotopic norepinephrine by cat tissues. *Nature* (London) 191:816, 1961.
175. Glowinski, J., and Axelrod, J. Effect of drugs on uptake, release and metabolism of H^3-norepinephrine in rat brain. *J. Pharmacol. & Exper. Therap.* 149:43–49, 1965.
176. Stein, L. Self-stimulation of brain and central stimulant action of amphetamine. *Federation Proc.* 23:836–850, 1964.

177. Gelder, M. G., and Vane, J. R. Interaction of effects of tyramine, amphetamine and reserpine in man. *Psychopharmacologia* 3:231–241, 1962.
178. Vane, J. R. Actions of sympathomimetic amines on tryptamine receptors. In Ciba Foundation. *Adrenergic Mechanisms (Papers and Discussions)*. Editor for British Pharmacological Society: J. R. Vane. Editors for Foundation: G. E. W. Wolstenholme and M. O'Connor. Boston: Little, Brown, 1961. (*Symposia, General Series.*) Pp. 356–372.
179. van Rossum, J. M., van der Schoot, J. B., and Hurkmans, J. A. Th. M. Mechanism of action of cocaine and amphetamine in brain. *Experientia* 18:229–231, 1962.
180. Smith, C. B. Effects of d-amphetamine upon brain amine content and locomotor activity of mice. *J. Pharmacol. & Exper. Therap.* 147:96–102, 1965.
181. Randrup, A., and Munkvad, I. Role of catecholamines in amphetamine excitatory response. *Nature* (London) 211:540, 1966.
182. Hanson, L. C. F. Evidence that central action of (+)-amphetamine is mediated via catecholamines. *Psychopharmacologia* 10:289–297, 1967.
183. Stein, L. Psychopharmacological substrates of mental depression. In *Anti-depressant Drugs: Proceedings. Organized by the Istituto di Ricerche Farmacologiche Mario Negri, Milan, April 25–27, 1966.* Edited by S. Garattini and M. N. G. Dukes. Amsterdam: Excerpta Medica, 1967. Pp. 130–140.
184. Sulser, F., Owens, M. L., Norvich, M. R., and Dingell, J. V. Relative role of storage and synthesis of brain norepinephrine in psychomotor stimulation evoked by amphetamine or by desipramine and tetrabenazine. *Psychopharmacologia* 12:322–332, 1968.
185. Moore, K. E., and Rech, R. H. Reversal of α-methyltyrosine-induced behavioural depression with dihydroxyphenylalanine and amphetamine. *J. Pharm. & Pharmacol.* 19:405–407, 1967.
186. McLean, J. R., and McCartney, M. Effect of D-amphetamine on rat brain noradrenaline and serotonin. *Proc. Soc. Exper. Biol. & Med.* 107:77–79, 1961.
187. Sanan, S., and Vogt, M. Effects of drugs on noradrenaline content of brain and peripheral tissues and its significance. *Brit. J. Pharmacol.* 18:109–127, 1962.
188. Moore, K. E., and Lariviere, E. W. Effects of D-amphetamine and restraint on content of norepinephrine and dopamine in rat brain. *Biochem. Pharmacol.* 12:1283–1288, 1963.
189. Carlton, P. L. Potentiation of behavioral effects of amphetamine by imipramine. *Psychopharmacologia* 2:364–376, 1961.
190. Weissman, A. Interaction effects of imipramine and d-amphetamine on non-discriminated avoidance. *Pharmacologist* 3 (2):60, Fall, 1961.
191. Scheckel, C. L., and Boff, E. Behavioral effects of interacting imipramine and other drugs with d-amphetamine, cocaine, and tetrabenazine. *Psychopharmacologia* 5:198–208, 1964.
192. Sulser, F., Owens, M. L., and Dingell, J. V. On mechanism of

amphetamine potentiation by desipramine (DMI). *Life Sc.* 5:2005–2010, 1966.

193. Valzelli, L., Consolo, S., and Morpurgo, C. Influence of imipramine-like drugs on metabolism of amphetamine. In *Anti-depressant Drugs: Proceedings. Organized by the Istituto di Ricerche Farmacologiche Mario Negri, Milan, April 25–27, 1966.* Edited by S. Garattini and M. N. G. Dukes. Amsterdam: Excerpta Medica, 1967. Pp. 61–69.
194. Trendelenburg, U. Supersensitivity caused by cocaine. *J. Pharmacol. & Exper. Therap.* 125:55–65, 1959.
195. Schildkraut, J. J., Schanberg, S. M., Breese, G. R., and Kopin, I. J. Norepinephrine metabolism and drugs used in affective disorders: Possible mechanism of action. *Am. J. Psychiat.* 124:600–608, 1967.
196. Shatalova, A. A., and Antonov, E. K. Content of adrenaline and noradrenaline in adrenal and brain tissues and in blood of rabbits in convulsive states. *Psychopharmacol. Abstr.* 1:341, 1961.
197. Breitner, C., Picchioni, A., and Chin, L. Neurohormone levels in brain after CNS stimulation including electrotherapy. *J. Neuropsychiat.* 5:153–158, 1964.
198. Garattini, S., and Valzelli, L. Serotonin and electroshock. In International Symposium on Psychotropic Drugs, Milan, 1957. *Psychotropic Drugs (Proceedings).* Edited by S. Garattini and V. Ghetti. Amsterdam: Elsevier, 1957. Pp. 428–436.
199. Garattini, S., Kato, R., Lamesta, L., and Valzelli, L. Electroshock, brain serotonin, and barbiturate narcosis. *Experientia* 16:156 1960.
200. Breitner, C., Picchioni, A., Chin, L., and Burton, L. E. Effect of electrostimulation on brain 5-hydroxytryptamine concentration. *Dis. Nerv. System* (Suppl.) 22 (4):93–96, 1961.
201. Bonnycastle, D. D., Giarman, N. J., and Paasonen, M. K. Anticonvulsant compounds and 5-hydroxytryptamine in rat brain. *Brit. J. Pharmacol.* 12:228–231, 1957.
202. Freedman, D. X. Psychotomimetic drugs and brain biogenic amines. *Am. J. Psychiat.* 119:843–850, 1963.
203. Maynert, E. W., and Levi, R. Stress-induced release of brain norepinephrine and its inhibition by drugs. *J. Pharmacol. & Exper. Therap.* 143:90–95, 1964.
204. Hinesley, R. K., Norton, J. A., and Aprison, M. H. Serotonin, norepinephrine and 3,4-dihydroxyphenylethylamine in rat brain parts following electroconvulsive shock. *J. Psychiat. Research* 6:143–152, 1968.
205. Kety, S. S., Javoy, F., Thierry, A. M., Julou, L., and Glowinski, J. Sustained effect of electroconvulsive shock on turnover of norepinephrine in central nervous system of rat. *Proc. Nat. Acad. Sc.* 58:1249–1254, 1967.
206. Thierry, A. M., Javoy, F., Glowinski, J., and Kety, S. S. Effects of stress on metabolism of norepinephrine, dopamine and serotonin in central nervous system of rat. I. Modifications of norepinephrine turnover. *J. Pharmacol. & Exper. Therap.* 163:163–171, 1968.
207. Engel, J., Hanson, L. C. F., Roos, B. E., and Strombergsson, L.

E. Effect of electroshock on dopamine metabolism in rat brain. *Psychopharmacologia* 13:140–144, 1968.

208. Cooper, A. J., Moir, A. T. B., and Guldberg, H. C. Effect of electroconvulsive shock on cerebral metabolism of dopamine and 5-hydroxytryptamine. *J. Pharm. & Pharmacol.* 20:729, 1968.

209. Schildkraut, J. J., Schanberg, S. M., and Kopin, I. J. Effects of lithium ion on H^3-norepinephrine metabolism in brain. *Life Sc.* 5:1479–1483, 1966.

210. Schildkraut, J. J., Logue, M. A., and Dodge, G. A. Effects of lithium salts on turnover and metabolism of norepinephrine in rat brain. *Psychopharmacologia* 14:135–141, 1969.

211. Haškovec, L., and Ryšánek, K. Die Wirkung von Lithium auf den Metabolismus der Katecholamine und Indolalkylamine beim Menschen. *Arzneimittel-Forsch.* 19:426–427, 1969.

212. Corrodi, H., Fuxe, K., Hökfelt, T., and Schou, M. Effect of lithium on cerebral monoamine neurons. *Psychopharmacologia* 11: 345–353, 1967.

213. Stern, D. M., Fieve, R., Neff, N., and Costa, E. Effect of lithium on turnover of brain and heart catecholamines. *Pharmacologist* 9:210, 1967.

214. Greenspan, K., Aranoff, M., and Bogdanski, D. F. Personal communication, 1968.

215. Colburn, R. W., Goodwin, F. K., Bunney, W. E., Jr., and Davis, J. M. Effect of lithium on uptake of noradrenaline by synaptosomes. *Nature* (London) 215:1395–1397, 1967.

216. Anumonye, A., Reading, H. W., Knight, F., and Ashcroft, G. W. Uric-acid metabolism in manic-depressive illness and during lithium therapy, *Lancet* 1:1290–1293, 1968.

217. Pollin, W., Cardon, P. V., Jr., and Kety, S. S. Effects of amino acid feedings in schizophrenic patients treated with iproniazid. *Science* 133:104, 1961.

218. Smith, B., and Prockop, D. J. Central-nervous-system effects of ingestion of L-trytophan by normal subjects. *New Eng. J. Med.* 267:1338–1341, 1962.

219. Coppen, A., Shaw, D. M., and Farrell, J. P. Potentiation of antidepressive effect of monoamine-oxidase inhibitor by tryptophan. *Lancet* 1:79–81, 1963.

220. Pare, C. M. B. Potentiation of monoamine-oxidase inhibitors by tryptophan. *Lancet* 2:527, 1963.

221. Coppen, A., Shaw, D. M., Herzberg, B., and Maggs, R. Tryptophan in treatment of depression. *Lancet* 2:1178–1180, 1967.

222. Kline, N. S., and Sacks, W. Relief of depression within one day using M.A.O. inhibitor and intravenous 5-HTP. *Am. J. Psychiat.* 120:274, 1963.

223. Kline, N. S., Sacks, W., and Simpson, G. M. Further studies on: one day treatment of depression with 5-HTP. *Am. J. Psychiat.* 121:379–381, 1964.

224. Pare, C. M. B., and Sandler, M. Clinical and biochemical study of trial of iproniazid in treatment of depression. *J. Neurol., Neurosurg. & Psychiat.* 22:247–251, 1959.

225. Klerman, G. L., Schildkraut, J. J., Hasenbush, L. L., Greenblatt, M., and Friend, D. G. Clinical experience with dihydroxyphenylalanine (DOPA) in depression. *J. Psychiat. Research* 1:289–297, 1963.
226. Cotzias, G. C., Van Woert, M. H., and Schiffer, L. M. Aromatic amino acids and modification of Parkinsonism. *New Eng. J. Med.* 276:374–379, 1967.
227. Turner, W. J., and Merlis, S. Clinical trial of pargyline and DOPA in psychotic subjects. *Dis. Nerv. System* 25:538–541, 1964.
228. Ingvarsson, C. G. Orientierende klinische Versuche zur Wirkung des Dioxyphenylalanins (l-Dopa) bei endogener Depression. *Arzneimittel-Forsch.* 15:849–852, 1965.
229. Matussek, N., Pohlmeier, H., and Ruther, E. Die Wirkung von Dopa auf gehemmte Depressionen. *Klin. Wchnschr.* 44:727, 1966.
230. Schildkraut, J. J., Klerman, G. L., Friend, D. G., and Greenblatt, M. Biochemical and pressor effects of oral D,L-dihydroxyphenylalanine in patients pretreated with antidepressant drugs. *Ann. New York Acad. Sc.* 107:1005–1015, 1963.
231. Pöldinger, W. Combined administration of desipramine and reserpine or tetrabenazine in depressive patients. *Psychopharmacologia* 4:308–310, 1963.
232. Dick, P., and Roch, P. Interaction of tricyclic antidepressants and tetrabenazine: Its clinical use and therapeutic results. In *Anti-depressant Drugs: Proceedings. Organized by the Istituto di Ricerche Farmacologiche Mario Negri, Milan, April 25–27, 1966.* Edited by S. Garattini and M. N. G. Dukes. Amsterdam: Excerpta Medica, 1967. Pp. 311–315.
233. Haškovec, L., and Ryšánek, K. Action of reserpine in imipramine-resistant depressive patients: Clinical and biochemical study. *Psychopharmacologia* 11:18–30, 1967.
234. Prange, A. J., Jr., Wilson, I. C., Rabon, A. M., and Lipton, M. A. Enhancement of imipramine antidepressant activity by thyroid hormone. *Am. J. Psychiat.* 126:457–469, 1969.
235. Lipton, M. A., Prange, A. J., Jr., Dairman, W., and Udenfriend, S. Increased rate of norepinephrine biosynthesis in hypothyroid rats. *Federation Proc.* 27:399, 1968.
236. Waldstein, S. S. Thyroid-catecholamine interrelations. *Ann. Rev. Med.* 17:123–132, 1966.
237. Dewhurst, W. G. Methysergide in mania. *Nature* (London) 219: 506, 1968.
238. Haškovec, L., and Souček, K. Trial of methysergide in mania. *Nature* (London) 219:507, 1968.
239. Dewhurst, W. G. Cerebral amines and behaviour. *Lancet* 2:514, 1968.
240. *Idem.* Cerebral amine functions in health and disease. In *Studies in Psychiatry.* Edited by M. Shepherd and D. L. Davies. London: Oxford University Press, 1968. Pp. 289–317.
241. Engelman, K., and Sjoerdsma, A. Inhibition of catecholamine biosynthesis in man. *Circulation Research* 18:104–109, 1966.
242. Engelman, K., Horwitz, D., Jéquier, E., and Sjoerdsma, A. Bio-

chemical and pharmacologic effects of α-methyltyrosine in man. *J. Clin. Investigation* 47:577–594, 1968.

243. Engelman, K., Lovenberg, W., and Sjoerdsma, A. Inhibition of serotonin synthesis by para-chlorophenylalanine in patients with carcinoid syndrome. *New Eng. J. Med.* 277:1103–1108, 1967.
244. Bueno, J. R., and Himwich, H. E. Dualistic approach to some biochemical problems in endogenous depressions. *Psychosomatics* 8:82–94, 1967.
245. Coppen, A. Biochemistry of affective disorders. *Brit. J. Psychiat.* 113:1237–1264, 1967.
246. Weil-Malherbe, H. Biochemistry of functional psychoses. *Advances in Enzymol.* 29:479–553, 1967.
247. Himwich, H. E. Indoleamines and depressions. In *Biochemistry, Schizophrenia and Affective Illnesses.* Edited by H. E. Himwich. Baltimore: Williams & Wilkins (in press).
248. Ström-Olsen, R., and Weil-Malherbe, H. Humoral changes in manic-depressive psychosis with particular reference to excretion of catechol amines in urine. *J. Ment. Sc.* 104:696–704, 1958.
249. Shinfuku, N., Omura, M., and Kayano, M. Catechol amine excretion in manic depressive psychosis. *Yonago acta med.* 5:109–114, 1961.

249a. Takahashi, R., Nagao, Y., Tsuchiya, K., Takamizawa, M., Kobayashi, T., Toru, M., Kobayashi, K., and Kariya, T. Catecholamine metabolism of manic-depressive illness. *J. Psychiat. Research* 6:185–199, 1968.

250. Sloane, R. B., Hughes, W., and Haust, H. L. Catecholamine excretion in manic-depressive and schizophrenic psychosis and its relationship to symptomatology. *Canad. Psychiat. A. J.* 11:6–19, 1966.
251. Bergsman, A. Urinary excretion of adrenaline and noradrenaline in some mental diseases: Clinical and experimental study. *Acta psychiat. & neurol. Scandinav.* 34 (Suppl. 133):5–107, 1959.
252. Curtis, G. C., Cleghorn, R. A., and Sourkes, T. L. Relationship between affect and excretion of adrenaline, noradrenaline, and 17-hydroxycortico-steroids. *J. Psychosom. Research* 4:176–184, 1960.
253. Greenspan, K., Schildkraut, J. J., Gordon, E. K., Baer, L., Aronoff, M. S., and Durell, J. Catecholamine metabolism in affective disorders. III. MHPG and other catecholamine metabolites in patients treated with lithium carbonate. *J. Psychiat. Research* 7:171–183, 1970.
254. Bunney, W. E., Jr., Davis, J. M., Weil-Malherbe, H., and Smith, E. R. B. Biochemical changes in psychotic depression: High norepinephrine levels in psychotic vs. neurotic depression. *Arch. Gen. Psychiat.* 16:448–460, 1967.
255. Nelson, G. N., Masuda, M., and Holmes, T. H. Correlation of behavior and catecholamine metabolite excretion. *Psychosom. Med.* 28:216–226, 1966.
256. Rosenblatt, S., and Chanley, J. D. Differences in metabolism of norepinephrine in depressions: Effects of various therapies. *Arch. Gen. Psychiat.* 13:495–502, 1965.

257. Greenspan, K., Schildkraut, J. J., Gordon, E. K., Levy, B., and Durell, J. Catecholamine metabolism in affective disorders. II. Norepinephrine, normetanephrine, epinephrine, metanephrine and VMA excretion in hypomanic patients. *Arch. Gen. Psychiat.* 21: 710–716, 1969.

258. Kärki, N. T. Urinary excretion of noradrenaline and adrenaline in different age groups, its diurnal variation and effect of muscular work on it. *Acta physiol. Scandinav.* 39 (Suppl. 132):5–96, 1956.

259. Weil-Malherbe, H., Axelrod, J., and Tomchick, R. Blood-brain barrier for adrenaline. *Science* 129:1226, 1959.

260. Glowinski, J., Kopin, I. J., and Axelrod, J. Metabolism of [H^3] norepinephrine in rat brain. *J. Neurochem.* 12:25–30, 1965.

261. Mass, J. W., and Landis, D. H. Technique for assaying kinetics of norepinephrine metabolism in central nervous system in vivo. *Psychosom. Med.* 28:247–256, 1966.

262. Schanberg, S. M., Breese, G. R., Schildkraut, J. J., Gordon, E. K., and Kopin, I. J. 3-Methoxy-4-hydroxyphenylglycol sulfate in brain and cerebrospinal fluid. *Biochem. Pharmacol.* 17:2006–2008, 1968.

263. Maas, J. W., Fawcett, J., and Dekirmenjian, H. 3-Methoxy-4-hydroxy phenylglycol (MHPG) excretion in depressive states: Pilot study. *Arch. Gen. Psychiat.* 19:129–134, 1968.

264. Rodnight, R. Body fluid indoles in mental illness. *Internat. Rev. Neurobiol.* 3:251–292, 1961.

265. Tissot, R. Connaissances expérimentales sur les monoamines et quelques syndromes psychiatriques. In *Monoamines et Système Nerveux Central: Symposium Bel-Air, Genève, Septembre 1961.* Edited by J. de Ajuriaguerra. Geneva: Georg, 1962. Pp. 169–207.

266. van Praag, H. M., and Leijnse, B. Die Bedeutung der Monoaminoxydasehemmung als antidepressives Prinzip. I. *Psychopharmacologia* 4:1–14, 1963.

267. Gayral, L., Bierer, R., and Delhom. A. L'excrétion urinaire de l'acide 5-hydroxy-indolacétique dans les dépressions et les mélancolies sous l'influence du traitement par les inhibiteurs de la monoamine-oxydase. In *Neuropsychopharmacology.* Edited by H. Brill et al. Amsterdam: Excerpta Medica, 1967. Pp. 339–342.

268. Crout, J. R., and Sjoerdsma. A. Clinical and laboratory significance of serotonin and catechol amines in bananas. *New Eng. J. Med.* 261:23–26, 1959.

269. Eccleston, D., Ashcroft, G. W., Moir, A. T. D., Parker-Rhodes, A., Lutz, W., and O'Mahoney, D. P. Comparison of 5-hydroxyindoles in various regions of dog brain and cerebrospinal fluid. *J. Neurochem.* 15: 947–957, 1968.

270. Ashcroft, G. W., Crawford, T. B. B., Eccleston, D., Sharman, D. F., MacDougall, E. J., Stanton, J. B., and Binns, J. K. 5-Hydroxyindole compounds in cerebrospinal fluid of patients with psychiatric or neurological diseases. *Lancet* 2:1049–1052, 1966.

271. Dencker, S. J., Malm, U., Roos, B. E., and Werdinius, B. Acid monoamine metabolites of cerebrospinal fluid in mental depression and mania. *J. Neurochem.* 13:1545–1548, 1966.

272. Fotherby, K., Ashcroft, G. W., Afflect, J. W., and Forrest, A. D. Studies on sodium transfer and 5-hydroxyindoles in depressive illness. *J. Neurosurg. & Psychiat.* 26:71–73, 1963.
273. Shaw, D. M., Camps, F. E., and Eccleston, E. G. 5-Hydroxytryptamine in hind-brain of depressive suicides. *Brit. J. Psychiat.* 113: 1407–1411, 1967.
274. Bourne, H. R., Bunney, W. E., Jr., Colburn, R. W., Davis, J. M., Davis, J. N., Shaw, D. M., and Coppen, A. J. Noradrenaline, 5-hydroxytryptamine and 5-hydroxyindoleacetic acid in hindbrains of suicidal patients. *Lancet* 2:805–808, 1968.
275. Coppen, A., Shaw, D. M., Malleson, A., Eccleston, E., and Gundy, G. Tryptamine metabolism in depression. *Brit. J. Psychiat.* 111: 993–998, 1965.
276. Coppen, A., Shaw, D. M., and Malleson, A. Changes in 5-hydroxytryptophan metabolism in depression. *Brit. J. Psychiat.* 111:105–107, 1965.
277. Cazzullo, C. L., Mangoni, A., and Mascherpa, G. Tryptophan metabolism in affective psychoses. *Brit. J. Psychiat.* 112:157–162, 1966.
278. Mandel, A. J. Some determinants of indole excretion in man. *Rec. Adv. Biol. Psychiat.* 5:237–256, 1963.
279. Lapin, I. P., and Oxenkrug, G. F. Intensification of the central serotoninergic processes as a possible determinant of the thymoleptic effect. *Lancet* 1:132–136, 1969.
280. Curzon, G. Metabolic changes in depression. *Lancet* 1:257, 1969.

INDEX

INDEX

Index